STRENGTH TRAINING FOR SENIORS

REWRITE YOUR FITNESS JOURNEY USING SIMPLE AND EFFECTIVE EXERCISES THAT HELP YOU IMPROVE BALANCE, BUILD CONFIDENCE AND BOOST ENERGY

LINDA ANDREWS

This book is dedicated to all seniors inspired to improve their overall health and well-being through strength training. I hope this book will provide you with the knowledge, skills, and motivation to embark on this journey and reap the rewards of a healthier, more active lifestyle. I wish you success in your pursuit!

Contents

Introduction

"Those who think they have no time for bodily exercise will sooner or later have to find time for illness."

— Edward Stanley

Did you know seniors who exercise frequently are less likely to rely on or depend on others?

Yes, exercise is an essential part of a healthy lifestyle throughout one's life, but for seniors, it's critical to staying independent and improving your health, among other benefits.

According to Harvard Medical School, regular exercise increases older adults' ability to walk, wash, cook, eat, dress, and use the lavatory. Practice is one of the finest ways for older persons to maintain independence if self-reliance is a priority.

Digging further, several researchers have discovered that many degenerative diseases and most general weaknesses accompanying aging are related to muscle mass and strength loss.

Although a certain amount of strength attenuation is inevitable, numerous studies have confirmed that older adults can maintain and regain muscle mass and strength at any age. Postmenopausal women, older men, and even nonagenarians have all improved their musculoskeletal structure and function through simple strength training programs.

Fortunately, the effective use of exercises makes it possible for older adults to practicalize strength training, enabling the weak to become strong, the sedentary active, and the disabled and dysfunctional capable and able. So if, at any point, you find yourself asking specific questions like:

How can I move around like I did when I was much younger and had a better balance?

Can we build strength after recovering from an injury?

How do I overcome this fear of falling and become flexible again as I used to be?

What can I do to reduce low-back pain and decrease arthritic discomfort?

What does it take to build muscular fitness and unlock higher levels of self-confidence?

You must start paying attention to your health and fitness lifestyle, especially strength training.

But sadly, no clearly defined exercise protocol exists for seniors' strength training.

Luckily, when you read this book to the end, you will discover how to start your fitness journey as you age. Oh yes! Whether you are in your 40s, 50s, 70s, or older, this book will show you simple strength training exercises to gain strength, improve balance and boost your confidence.

Despite being sidelined with a back injury in my 50s, I never used that as an excuse or belittled myself. My intense desire to find alternative ways to heal, rather than prescribed medicine, led to immersing myself in studying fitness and general well-being.

Thanks to my love for reading and researching, I burnt the midnight candle studying several fitness guides, practicalizing all I studied and learned from my successes and failures. It was a journey of self-discovery.

My recovery took less than two years. I started with small steps using a cane and eventually moved into exercising. I kept at it until I could walk miles around my family. It was a roller coaster experience, but I learned that all is not lost as we age.

Because our biology changes as we age, seniors have different motivations for staying fit than younger generations. Though physical fitness benefits people of all ages, the health benefits that physically active seniors enjoy are more noticeable. According to doctors and academics, elders should be as active as possible without overdoing it. Exercise helps older folks have a longer, healthier, and more joyful life.

Though it may appear counterintuitive, being idle causes fatigue, while being active provides more incredible energy. Endorphins, crucial neurotransmitters connected to pain relief and a sensation of well-being, are released in response to any amount of exercise. Endorphins fight stress hormones, support proper sleep, and help you feel alive and active.

Falling is a much bigger deal for older adults than younger ones. According to the National Council of Aging, every 11 seconds, an older adult is admitted to the emergency room for a fall-related injury, and an older adult dies from a fall every 19 minutes. Even though no two falls are unique and avoiding falls is a complex process, regular exercise reduces the probability of falling by 23%.

Strength training helps to reduce the risk of falling as we age by improving balance, coordination, and flexibility. Strength training can also increase muscle strength, which helps to support the joints, improving stability, and reducing the risk of falls. Additionally, strength training can help improve bone density, reducing the risk of fractures from falls. Finally, strength training can help to improve posture, which can help to reduce the risk of falls due to impaired balance.

Adopting a more active lifestyle also helps prevent and counteract common, often deadly diseases among older adults like heart disease, osteoporosis, depression, and diabetes. And according to a research study from NCBI, older adults who exercise regularly have improved cognitive health, especially since the body and the mind work closely together.

I am writing this book because I have been through the "Oh My Goodness" process of never feeling like I could move again, slowly coming to terms with my injury, starting to move, and finally feeling back to normal.

All of my knowledge and experiences are what I have poured into this book, which extensively addresses the subject of fitness and strength training exercises for seniors.

Strength Training for Seniors will teach you to rewrite your fitness and health journey using the tools and resources I have provided to gain the benefits of strength training. Ultimately, you will understand all it takes to live a long and healthy life and why you don't even have to age.

I hope you opened this book because you have at least a vague interest in health, fitness, and exercise, but like so many seniors before you, you have yet to learn how to start. See this book as your fitness compass. It will help you understand strength training and learn its nitty-gritty.

Strength, instead of weakness, is the capacity to defy gravity and resistance and move with vitality and vigor. Strength is the energy that allows us to produce force, to conduct expert and strong motions, instead of giving way, yielding, crumbling, and falling.

Strength is the impulse, dynamics, and momentum that drives the human body's ability to act with force and energy. We would decay, succumb, crumble, and fail if we lacked sufficient strength. We wouldn't be able to do any activities that keep us healthy and fit as adults if we didn't have strength.

In choosing to read this guide, you have taken the right step in rewriting your fitness journey, building greater strength, and enjoying lifelong vitality. I wrote this book for you—the senior who wants to grow healthier, stronger, more active, and more independent.

You could be inactive or only moderately active right now. Regular exercise benefits your health and well-being, and you wish to begin a physical activity program. However, you may need more information. Perhaps you are anxious that physical activity will be unsafe due to age or health issues. You may need help finding or sticking with an appropriate program.

Strength Training for Seniors offers you safe, simple, and highly effective exercise activities based on the principles of strength training. A successful strength training program can make the difference between older adults with low strength levels who endure a sedentary existence and those with high strength levels who enjoy a physically active lifestyle. The information in this guide will enhance your knowledge of strength training and enable you to live a healthy lifestyle as you age.

Strength training as we age is important because it helps to maintain and improve physical strength, endurance, and mobility. It also helps to reduce the risk of injury and improve overall health. Benefits include increased bone density, improved posture, balance, and coordination, increased muscle mass and strength, joint flexibility and mobility, and cardiovascular health. It can also help to increase metabolism, which can help with weight management. Finally, strength training can help to improve mental health and reduce the risk of depression.

While changes like reduced bone mass and muscle are unavoidable as we grow older, maintaining your strength and being active can prevent them to an extent. And so, my hope for you is that this book inspires you to train safely and effectively so you gain more strength and enjoy a practical, no-nonsense approach to fitness training.

I want to thank all those who have received and read this book. Once you have finished reading, I am asking for you to please leave a kind review. I would love to hear your feedback!

Are you feeling excited already?

Well, then, let's get started!

Chapter 1: Why Strength Training Is Important

"When it comes to health and well-being, regular exercise is about as close to a magic potion as possible."

– Tich Nhat Hanh

Do you want to live forever?

Young Tithonus, son of King Laomedon and lover of Eos, goddess of dawn, wanted to live forever. In mythical times, this was a privilege reserved for the dwellers of Mount Olympus, also known as the gods!

The goddess Eos had fallen in love with the young prince. As a result, she took him from his father's house as her husband. She wanted Tithonus to be with her forever, but he was a mortal. And for a man to be granted immortality, he needed special permission from Zeus, the king of the gods.

One day, the goddess of dawn approached Zeus and asked him to make her lover immortal, and Zeus granted the request. Indeed, her lover, Tithonus, lived forever, but old age came upon him, and he could not move his limbs. He lost all his strength and control of his faculties. Some versions of the story claimed he turned into a Cicada to beg for death.

Eos surely did not wish for her lover to suffer, but she had asked for the wrong thing. An ideal request would be in line with the lyrics of the 1984 classic by Alphaville, "Forever Young." Youthfulness would have made Tithonus's immortality enjoyable, as the pair would have lived every day in their prime lives.

Old age has many benefits, including wisdom and an understanding of life's ever-changing patterns and trends. It also grants one a wealth of experience and mental strength but often leaves one needing more physical strength. As people age, they notice a significant decline in physical attributes, such as strength, speed, tolerance, and recovery time. Thus, they will find specific physical tasks more challenging and complain more about aches after extended physical activity.

A professional soccer player once lamented, saying, "I'm no longer twenty-two; my body can't do things that it used to."

This happens because as human beings grow, the body changes. A newborn human has an average height of nineteen to twenty inches, with tiny hands and legs dependent on their parents for everything. Gradually, the baby grows, and its body changes. At four, kids have an average height of forty inches and can do simple tasks without assistance. At puberty, the body changes significantly for children of both sexes. Girls notice physical and physiological changes like the growth of breasts and menstruation, among other things, while boys become taller and stronger with firmer muscles and stronger bones.

Human beings continue to grow in strength and reach peak physical health in their thirties. And this growth follows an upward trajectory until they become seniors. In old age, one becomes progressively weaker because aging affects body support structures like bones, joints, and muscles.

"Old age grants one a wealth of experience and mental strength but often leaves one lacking physical strength."

How Aging Affects Your Bones, Joints, and Muscles

The human skeleton is the internal framework of the human body. It contains around 270 bones at birth, which reduces to 206 after some bones have fused by adulthood, and connective tissues like cartilage, tendons, and ligaments.

Bones, muscles, and joints are the major parts of the human musculoskeletal system and are assisted by the connective tissues. Together, they maintain our primary physical attributes.

A joint is an area where two or more bones meet. The cartilage cushions bones inside joints and also connect bones. Ligaments are strong bands of tissues that join bones and help the joints remain strong. Finally, tendons contain vital connective tissues that connect muscles to bones. Together, they make up the human skeleton.

Bones store minerals like calcium and phosphorus and contain bone marrow that produces blood cells. There are thirty-three bones in the vertebral column, which is the body's central support, and specific gel-like structures called discs separate these bones from one another.

Skeletal muscles are muscles that are controlled voluntarily. They run across bones, passing at least one joint in their way, and can be strengthened by performing physical activities.

These structures enable the skeleton to carry out its functions. The human frame has six primary functions, and three of them help human beings be physically active. They are support, movement, and protection.

- **Support:** The human skeleton supports the body and maintains its shape. For example, the lungs will collapse without the help of the rib cages, costal cartilage, and intercostal muscles.

- **Movement:** Skeletal muscles attached to the bones enable movement. Muscles, bones, and joints, coordinated by the nervous system, make it possible for human beings to move.

- **Protection:** The skeleton protects vital organs from damage. The skull keeps the brain safe, while the vertebrae keep the spinal cord safe.

However, as humans age, it becomes more difficult for the skeleton to carry out its functions because the bones and muscles lose features that make them more effective in a human's youth.

How Aging Affects the Bones

The bones lose density or mass as you near old age. The bones attain maximum density at age twenty-one and stay stable between ages twenty-five and fifty. After age fifty, bones break down faster than they form, and bone loss increases, particularly in women undergoing menopause. The bone also loses essential nutrients during this phase, like calcium.

Furthermore, the body's trunk becomes shorter as the disks between the vertebrae bones lose fluids and become thin. The vertebrae also lose nutrients, and bones become leaner as a result—the vertebral column curves and compresses, which makes the body seem shorter.

The bones of the arms and legs lose nutrients and become weaker but rarely change in length. The bones become brittle and more likely to break, and height decreases as the trunk and spine shorten.

How Aging Affects the Joints

As people age. their joints lose flexibility, and their body fluids reduce. The joints around their knees and hips may also lose cartilage. The fingers also lose cartilage, causing the bones to thicken. The joint's weakening can lead to swelling, pain, and stiffness. And almost all older people feel the effects of aging on their joints.

Their posture changes, then their movement and gait slow and become unsteady. Arthritis is the most common problem of the joint, and most older adults develop this problem.

How Aging Affects the Muscles

Fat lodges in muscle tissues as humans age, and the muscle fibers start to shrink. The rate of tissue replacement also slows, and tough fibrous tissues replace lost muscle tissues. The result could make a person look thin and bony. Then, the body loses strength and endurance as muscles are lost.

Muscles lose their ability to contract and may become rigid as humans age. Some older people may experience involuntary movements and muscle tremors.

The loss of muscle mass reduces strength and endurance, making movement more challenging.

As your aging progresses, your loved ones will fearfully watch these changes happen in real-time. You will feel your body get weaker and worry that you can't do the things you could typically do. You will also fear that these changes may make you dependent; these are all legitimate fears, such as being neglected by their families when these issues surface. Those considered difficult by their loved ones are brought to older people's homes with overworked staff. However, there are better situations than this. Old age should be a time to enjoy the company of your children and grandchildren and everything you have gathered.

The good news is you don't have to grow old worrying about these issues if you prepare ahead. In this chapter, you will learn about steps to remain healthy as you age.

Staying Healthy in Old Age

Like nectar in Greek mythology, Ambrosia was a source of sustenance for the ancient Greek gods. They all remained immortal and maintained their youthfulness by consuming Ambrosia. Hera, the wife of Zeus, ate Ambrosia, which cleansed all defects from her skin. Also, with Ambrosia, Athena stripped away the effects of years from Penelope as she prepared her for her suitors.

As mortals, there is no particular food or nectar to help us maintain the strength and activeness of our youth. Still, there are several ways to support our physical health.

Seniors can maintain their health by changing habits and other aspects of their lifestyle to meet the demands of old age. And here are some ways they can do this:

Strength Training

The muscles and other structures of the skeletal system are strengthened by constant motion and physical activity. As you grow older, losing energy and strength is inevitable. You would likely face physical challenges if you led a sedentary life as a younger person. However, even those who were active in their youth can't outrun the passing of time and the changes it brings.

Even so, it is possible to slow down aging effects and maintain relative health by doing strength training. Strength training refers to exercises to strengthen your bones and muscles and maintain your physical health in old age. With strength training, you can build your strength, improve your balance and coordination, and reduce the risks of falling. You can avoid the loss of bone density that comes with old age and remain independent for as long as you want. Strength training also helps to lessen the effects of illnesses like arthritis, osteoporosis, etc. Furthermore, it reduces joint pain and stiffness and increases the body's metabolism to burn fat faster.

Research shows that strength training can also help to maintain mental and emotional well-being. Regular exercise helps you sleep better, reduce depression and improve your self-esteem.

If you were a Greek god or goddess, strength training is your Ambrosia.

However, before exercising, you should reach out to your doctor to ensure it is safe. And if they say it's safe for you, you have no excuses. So get to work today and get fit!

Proper Nutrition

One of the secrets of healthy living, regardless of age, is eating properly. Some describe eating properly as following all the rules of acceptable dining etiquette, but in this context, it means eating highly nutritious food—a balanced diet. A balanced diet provides the body with all essential nutrients, like proteins, vitamins, fibers, carbohydrates for energy, and fluids for osmoregulation.

Parents constantly remind their kids to eat their veggies whether or not they like them. Society generally focuses on the nutritional demands of children since their growth is essential to the survival of our species. However, while this is a good cause, we often focus so much on it that we need to pay attention to the needs of seniors.

Humans are born with about 10,000 taste buds, working with our sense of smell to give us an idea of our environment. However, your ability to taste and smell worsen with age. Most people lose some of their taste buds between ages forty and fifty. And at age sixty, it becomes more difficult to decipher what tastes sweet, sour, or bitter.

Losing one's sense of taste can sometimes lead to a loss of appetite. Our sense of taste makes food enjoyable, so when we lose it, we may lose interest in food. The loss of taste buds can also make one seek flavor from unhealthy sources, which could lead to weight gain and obesity.

Food is essential for human sustenance, and eating healthy amounts with the right nutrient proportions can help improve your health. Proper nutrition can help to prevent diseases like high blood pressure, type 2 diabetes, and some heart diseases associated with old age.

Proper nutrition requires paying attention to your nutritional needs. This requires you to consider your bodily changes and any existing health issues and set a plan based on your assessment.

Older people often eat less protein than required, which is unhealthy. Proteins help prevent muscle mass loss and maintain one's physical health. So as you grow older, fortify your diet with protein sources like dairy, peas, beans, and lentils, which provide other nutrients like vitamins D and B12. Staying hydrated may also require effort because you may feel less thirsty as you grow older. You can stay hydrated by drinking water, or for a little twist, add lemon to your water.

The bones and muscles are not the only parts of the body that decline with age; the brain also feels the impact of aging. Research has shown that the brain loses volume and weight at a rate of 5% per decade after age forty. However, the rate increases after age seventy. The brain loses nerve cells, which is linked to the shrinking of the gray matter. The physical changes that occur in the brain have cognitive ramifications, but the cognitive ability most affected by old age is memory. There are four classes of memory:

- Episodic memory

- Semantic memory

- Procedural memory

- Working memory

While all four classes of memory change as we age, episodic and semantic memories are the two that are significantly affected by age. Episodic memory is where information is retained. It connects to a place or time and how the data was acquired. An example of this is your first day at a new job or the first time you met a friend. This memory declines from age forty-five and advances well into old age. The loss is more severe with Alzheimer's disease.

Semantic memory, however, is related to the meanings of words and concepts and their use in daily living. This memory improves from the median age to the young-old but declines at more advanced ages.

You can slow the brain's decline rate by doing mental exercises. Constant use of the brain keeps it sharp and active. To remain mentally alert, seniors can play memory or word games and do puzzles as a recreation. Ultimately, this will keep them happy and maintain the brain's health.

Mental exercises keep the brain healthy enough to send instructions to other body parts. However, this is only possible if other body parts are fit enough to carry out these instructions. So to maintain your independence in old age, the bones and muscles in your limbs must remain strong, which is why strength training is essential.

Benefits of Strength Training

Strength training involves performing physical exercises to improve strength and endurance. It consists of a variety of training methods like bodyweight exercises and plyometrics.

Strength training is suitable for people of all ages but becomes more critical when the body becomes weaker in old age.

Here are some ways strength training helps to keep you healthy;

****Muscle strengthening**

Research has shown that even a short strength training program can help to rebuild lost muscle tissues in people between the ages of fifty and ninety. Strength training for three to four months helps in the gaining of muscles. It also helps to strengthen muscles that have weakened due to inactivity. Muscle cells subjected to regular strength training combined with proper protein intake undergo hypertrophy or enlargement of cells in response to the activity, which helps strengthen the muscles and their interaction with the nervous system.

****Improved balance, posture, mobility, and injury prevention**

Strength training helps to prevent the change in gait and posture that comes with old age. Naturally, a lack of regular physical activity worsens poor posture. Poor posture also indicates that a person has weak core muscles.

However, strength training awakens muscle cells and keeps the body lean, which helps to improve gait and balance. Strength training also helps prevent falls or unsteady injuries, which are common among older adults. It makes movement more manageable and helps maintain a good fitness level.

****Increased energy and endurance**

Strength training helps to boost energy and keep you active. It also causes the body to produce energy and nutrients for the structures of the cardiovascular system. With a stronger heart and lungs, the body can achieve more daily. Strength training also helps to improve bone and muscle capacity to take tension. Furthermore, it energizes and sustains you to carry out your daily activities, allowing you to maintain your independence.

**Improved metabolism and weight management

One of the essential health benefits of strength training is that it boosts your metabolism. Metabolism breaks down food into usable energy. However, when one consumes more calories than the body can burn, it results in weight gain. Unfortunately, our body's metabolism slows down as we age. And as physical activity reduces in old age, fat and calorie accumulation occurs.

Strength training is vital at this stage of life as it increases the fat and calorie expenditure rate, which helps you manage your weight. It improves body metabolism and helps your body efficiently maintain healthy fat levels.

**Stronger bones

Strength training helps to improve bone density and strength in old age. It also induces osteoblasts (bone-forming cells) production, which helps improve bone mass. In older women, strength training helps to prevent osteoporosis, which can lead to fractures. It increases mineral density in the bones, making them resistant to tension and shock.

**Quicker recovery

Physical activity becomes more challenging in old age. Walking a certain distance or doing other physical activities in old age requires more energy than in youth. It takes longer to recover after engaging in physical activities. Strength training helps to improve your endurance and recover from physical activities quicker. Ultimately, recovery is easier and faster when you have stronger bones, muscles, lungs, and heart.

**Improved mental health

Strength training improves your physical condition, which helps to boost self-esteem. Stress and anxiety are two of the most significant contributors to mental health deterioration. Fortunately, strength training can help you release tension and clear your headspace. It can also reduce depression and help you sleep better at night.

****Improved cognitive functions**

By reducing stress and anxiety, strength training makes it easier for the brain to focus on essential functions. Studies have shown that physical activity helps to improve memory, problem-solving skills, and emotional balance. Strength training puts all body parts in the best condition to perform their functions, making you more effective in old age.

Other benefits of strength training are as follows:

- Improved digestion

- Hormonal balance

- Disease prevention

- Blood pressure stability

- Blood sugar regulation

Strength training helps you age with grace and strength. It is a challenging journey that requires focus, dedication, commitment, and time. Strength training also improves the general quality of life, which is very important in old age.

Each chapter of this book guides you through this journey and makes you a stronger senior. If you need information and knowledge on the many demands of strength training, keep reading. The next chapter will guide you on how to begin your strength training.

Chapter 2: Starting Your Fitness Journey

"The journey of a thousand miles begins with one step."

– Lao Tzu

Everyone has goals and ambitions, and we have a century's worth of people who set and achieve goals. All these people will tell you one thing: achieving success begins by taking a single step. Although this seems simple, getting yourself to start is the most challenging aspect of any process. This is a broad experience, and a woman called Stephanie knows all about it.

Stephanie struggled to start her fitness journey. From a very young age, she was no fan of sports or physical exercise. She also paid no attention to her diet; for instance, she ate excess sugar, and eventually, her habits caught up with her. Stephanie weighed 300 pounds, which was her wake-up call. She decided one day to change her diet, and she did. First, she stopped drinking soda and beer and gave up chocolates which helped her lose fifty pounds, but that was not enough. She needed to start exercising. At first, she struggled to decide what schedule to follow, then put off working out for months.

However, everything changed when Stephanie decided to take a walk one day. She walked until she came upon a tennis court and decided to run its length on one side. Then decided to run one side and another, then around the full court. And since then, she has never looked back. A few months later, she ran her first mile and has steadily progressed in her fitness journey.

Stephanie realized after she started that getting fit wasn't as hard as she made it look, which is valid for all human endeavors. The longer you wait, the more complicated everything seems.

Like Stephanie, you have made the first step by reading this book. Having adequate knowledge of whatever you commit yourself to is an excellent way to start and a guarantee that you will continue halfway through; fortunately, this book provides all that. A sufficient understanding of this activity helps prepare the mind for the task ahead and will guide you through each step of the process.

In this chapter, we will discuss the importance of your mindset and how you can stay motivated.

The Importance of Your Mindset

People are only as good, strong, or effective as they think. Whether an individual succeeds or fails is based on their mindset.

Years of extensive psychological research show that your mindset can influence real-life outcomes. Furthermore, your attitude can affect your physical and mental health and make you more effective.

A positive mindset helps you break down complex situations and set expectations. It also forms the basis for your belief system that guides your decision-making process and outlook on life. The average human reaction to having a deadly disease is to be sad or depressed; some may even begin to put their affairs in order. Then again, some see it as another obstacle to scale through and an opportunity to become stronger. Nonetheless, the difference between this set of people is their mindset.

A 2012 study shows how having different mindsets in a particular situation can lead to different outcomes. The participants were people who experienced high levels of stress. The study showed that a high-stress level increases the risk of death, but only in those who believed stress is harmful. Those who experienced high-stress levels but didn't consider it dangerous had no increased risk of death. This study is evidence that your mindset has real-life implications.

Mindsets can be placed in two categories: fixed and growth.

People with fixed mindsets believe their habits and attitudes are fixed and unchangeable. This kind of mindset can be harmful and often lead to depression. A fixed mindset causes one to see mistakes as inherent flaws and leaves little room for self-betterment.

On the other hand, those with a growth mentality believe that their habits and attitude are not fixed and can be changed. They think that they can improve and are always motivated to get better. Their attitude to mistakes and setbacks is more forgiving. Also, they are less afraid of errors, enabling them to take risks that can lead to great success. Warren Buffet is one of the most famous adopters of the growth mindset. His mindset helps him go to bed every night better than he was the previous night.

The journey of physical fitness is one of self-improvement, which is only possible with the right mindset. One of the first steps toward optimum physical health in old age is acknowledging the work required and believing you can do it. Even in the prime of life, getting fit is a challenging commitment to make. However, assuming you can do it keeps you going on tough days.

Adopting the right mindset begins by asking yourself what you hope to achieve in your fitness journey. Ask yourself the question, "Why am I working out?"

As you discover, your "why" is to write down your short-term and long-term goals. Let them guide your schedule. Knowing your "why" is crucial as it guides you through each step. It also provides an avenue to monitor your progress and keeps you motivated.

"People with a growth mindset believe that their attitudes and habits can be changed. They think they can improve and are always motivated to improve."

Staying Motivated

Staying in shape requires a high level of commitment and mental strength that can be too demanding sometimes. It requires you to get up every day and intentionally put your body through stress to become stronger. You will inevitably feel tired or weak on some days. And on such days, you will require a clutch to keep you going.

Famous film star Dwayne Johnson is well known for his physique. He achieved his superb form by committing himself to an intense workout schedule. Despite already looking great, Johnson still subjects himself to rigorous strength training and approaches it daily with a positive mindset. However, even the fittest people have days when they feel unmotivated. Johnson once shared how he deals with such days while interacting with fans on his social media. When preparing to work out after a long day of shooting movies and doing media runs, an internal conversation occurs where he tries to convince himself to push through the tiredness. Finding motivation, he remembers his early days when he struggled financially and how that all changed by working hard, even when he felt weak or tired. He draws strength from his many life experiences.

Most people have fewer experiences to draw strength from than Dwayne Johnson or are more advanced in age, but they can find other ways to stay motivated. Here are some ways to stay motivated:

****Find ways to make exercise fun**

One way to stay motivated is to make working out an activity to look forward to doing. Making your workout sessions fun keeps you motivated. Mixing up the schedule and trying new exercises and equipment can make your sessions more fun. Doing the same daily routine can get boring and make you less motivated, so remember to change it. You can also keep the sessions fun by changing the intensity of your exercises. You can do high-intensity workouts for a certain period, then rest and go more slowly.

****Make working out a social activity**

Another way to stay motivated is to make working out a social activity. You can work out alone, but like everything on earth, workouts are more fun with friends. You can work out at home, but find time during the week to exercise with your friends, children, or grandchildren in the gym or at home. That way, you will strengthen each other's resolve when the going gets tough. You could also join a dance class.

****Fit exercise into your daily schedule**

Work can get overwhelming, making it challenging to find time to exercise, but you must find ways to plan around it. For instance, you could work out very early in the morning or after work at night. Find ways to fit exercise into your daily plan and miss no days. You can also find ways to exercise at work by remaining active. Use the stairs instead of the elevator, park farther from your work, and walk the distance. You could use the gym at your workplace or join its fitness network if there is one.

****Track your progress**

The best way to stay motivated is to see how far you have come from your starting point. Tracking your progress and celebrating your little wins helps you know that exercise is not a waste of time and effort and motivates you to keep it up. Achieving short-term goals gives you the confidence to tackle long-term goals and achieve more success. So remember to update your exercise plans as you accomplish your goals.

Before starting your fitness journey, it is wise to set goals for yourself, as this can help you stay focused. A proven framework for setting goals is to follow the old acronym SMART.

Setting SMART Goals

SMART goals are Specific, Measurable, Achievable, Real, and Timely. A specific goal is clear, concise, and focused on achieving a set objective. A measurable goal has a clear way of tracking its progress and accomplishments. An achievable goal may be challenging but is within your capacity to attain. A basic plan aligns with your present needs and is worth the effort. A timely goal helps to set deadlines for each step of the process and follows specific deadlines.

A SMART goal has all elements of a successful plan and leaves room for improvement. After six months or a year following the SMART framework, you can monitor your progress and fix your deficient areas.

Here is how to set SMART goals:

1. **Be specific** (this is your who, what, where, when, and why of your journey)

Setting a smart goal requires you first to find your "why." You start by deciding what you hope to achieve by exercising. Most people lose motivation after a few weeks or months because they failed to specify their wants. They start with only a general idea of what they hope to achieve, which makes them unprepared for the demands of a new lifestyle.

The general idea may be to get fit or get healthier but go one step further and specify which body parts need extra attention. If you have a genetic disposition for certain illnesses in old age, your goal could be to work hard to avoid disease in that body part. Or you could define what getting healthier means to you. For example, if you are overweight, a SMART goal will be to lose five pounds in one month.

Below are other examples of specific fitness goals:

- **Increasing the number of miles you can run**

- Building stronger bones and muscles.

- Cutting sugar out of your diet.

2. Assess the cost (this is measurable: how many goals and to track your progress)

After setting your specific goal, the next step is to assess the cost of achieving it and decide if it is realistic. If the goal is to lose an exact weight in a particular time frame, you must check to see what that will demand from you. Usually, losing weight will require changing your diet and replacing junk with vegetables. You may need the help of a nutritionist for this, and it should be considered part of your overall plan.

It will also require you to engage in specific exercises, which may require changing your daily schedule. You may have to wake up earlier every day or cut down on time allocated to other activities to accommodate the new movement. But whatever you do, you must carefully assess each demand and ensure you can meet them.

3. Set realistic deadlines (is this achievable; is this attainable; are your goals realistic)

After deciding that you can meet the demands of your new goal, set a deadline for yourself. This will help you to maintain discipline and motivation. An ideal deadline will challenge you without overextending you, or you may burn out. Building a new house can be done in a year, while losing weight or building stronger muscles can be achieved in less time. Challenge yourself but remain gracious. Consider the free time available during the day and see how much you can spare for your fitness goals.

Make sure you set criteria for monitoring your progress. You will know when you need to catch up or if you are overachieving.

4. Prepare for obstacles (reality check; is it worth it; are you prepared to do it)

After setting a framework to monitor your progress, the next task is to think of potential obstacles and ways to avoid them. Getting fit is challenging, and you will likely encounter problems as you progress. To avoid getting discouraged, you must prepare for each of them ahead of time.

The likely difficulties you may face in your fitness journey are accessing a gym or an instructor, getting equipment, getting injured, or feeling unwilling to exercise. Prepare ahead for them, and your chances of success become better.

5. Timely (what can you achieve today, in a week, in a month. and so on)

Once you set your goal, you must have realistic timing. If you do not have a reasonable time frame, you will not likely succeed. Give yourself a target date for reaching each goal. Ask yourself specific questions about the goal deadline and what can be accomplished. If your goal will take three months to complete, break it down into small goals throughout your journey. Using time constraints also creates a sense of urgency.

- **Note:** A goal is only SMART if you factor in your limitations. You must consider your strengths and weaknesses through every step of the process, or you may fail. So speak to your doctor and create fitness goals that will make you healthier without endangering you.

Setting SMART goals is essential and effective, but you can only achieve them with the right mindset and actions.

Your fitness journey will require you to make significant changes to your lifestyle. But first, you will have to shed habits that make you unhealthy and adopt better practices.

Eliminating Bad Habits

Forming new habits is difficult after a certain age, but it is necessary if you want to age gracefully. When you were younger, you could have gotten away with an unhealthy diet or sleep pattern, but the effects of a poor diet or sleeping habits are more intense when you are older. You must identify and remove these bad habits at the start of your fitness journey.

Breaking your bad habits requires you first to identify your triggers. An example of a bad habit that harms your health is staying up late. However, the first step to breaking such a habit is determining its cause.

Track this habit for a few days and pick out patterns that lead to sleeping late. This process will help you know if your late nights are caused by work or watching TV during late hours. After identifying the triggers, work on eliminating them. For instance, you could turn off your TV at 8 p.m. or not come home with any work.

Eliminating bad habits is easier when you have the support of a friend or a family member. Your friend or family member can help you stay disciplined when you are weak. They can hold you accountable and create an environment free of triggers to make the process more manageable.

One thing that helps when eliminating a bad habit is replacing it with a different one. You are more likely to fall back into your harmful pattern if you don't replace the void with something. For instance, someone trying to stop eating candy can break the bad habit and pick up fruit instead of candy when they crave it. You can acquire a new pattern using the 3-Rs principle.

The three Rs are reminders, routine, and reward.

- Reminder refers to what triggers a habit. It could be a craving or a feeling like hunger or stress. This feeling often starts a particular action.

- Routine refers to the actions associated with a trigger. For example, you always eat cake or chocolate when stressed. In that case, your brain will recognize the pattern and associate cake with relieving stress.

- The reward is what makes a habit stick. The pleasure you get from an action causes a chemical reaction in your brain that makes you want to repeat said action. For example, if you eat cake to relieve stress, your brain will release dopamine every time you do. This hormone reminds you to eat cake whenever you feel stressed, which is how you form that habit.

By understanding this, you can eliminate and replace bad habits with good ones. You can trick your brain into creating new patterns by changing your response to a trigger. Instead of satisfying the urge, do something different and shock the system. Gradually, your brain will recognize the new pattern and reward the new habit.

It is easy to fall back on familiar patterns, so you must remember to stick to your new routines. Ask friends to remind you, set reminders on your phone and TV, and keep the goal at the back of your mind. Setbacks are inevitable, but they don't make you weak. So be gracious to yourself and leave room for mistakes, as they are necessary for growth.

Start with little habits before attempting the bigger ones. Trying to break all bad habits at once will only lead to failure. So start easy and let the small wins motivate you to tackle more significant challenges.

Examples of habits to replace bad ones are adopting a healthy diet, sleeping and rising early, taking leisure walks, etc.

Remember to reward yourself for each success. Celebrate your small wins and cherish them as part of the journey. Also, share each breakthrough with your loved ones. That way, the habits will stick.

As you prepare to start your fitness journey, after adopting the right mentality and setting realistic goals, buy equipment for your exercises.

Some of the types of equipment you need are as follows:

- Strong chairs

- Good shoes with support

- Two-, three-, five-, and eight-pound dumbbells for men and women

- Two-, three-, five-, and eight-pound ankle weights for men and women

Your journey toward physical fitness has finally started, as this chapter has equipped you with the knowledge required to start. Adopt a positive mindset and let it affect all areas of your life. Next, accept that your bad habits are changeable and break them. Then, set SMART goals and celebrate each win. Armed with such knowledge, you are finally ready to become fit.

After years of unuse, a machine usually requires warming up before intense work to avoid breakdown. The body is similar to a machine, which requires warming up before physical activity after years of being sedentary. In the next chapter, your journey begins with learning how to warm up the body.

Chapter 3: Warming Up!

"P*eople think I can just walk out and shoot 75 without taking a warm-up shot. But believe me; it's not that easy."*

– Jim Nantz

How would you feel if someone crept up behind you and shouted, "Hell yes," in your ear? Awkward, right?

Well, that's what you do to your heart and muscles when exercising without warming up first. It helps prepare your body safely and effectively for rigorous activities.

A warm-up is a group of exercises one performs just before an activity, which helps the person's body adjust from a state of rest to exercise. It is essential to every physical activity or sports session, not just strength training, as it prepares the body appropriately for a workout.

Going straight into push-ups or squats on a cold day and then collapsing immediately is not recommended! Not only are painful muscle strains likely to follow, but the experience might be uncomfortable or even distressing for seniors. Aching muscles may be a painful reminder of the event for several days afterward.

Easing into strength training exercises ensures that the activity experience is more comfortable and that there is less likelihood of any injury. Safe involvement in an enjoyable movement is vital to promote long-term participation in physical activities. In contrast, uncomfortable and painful exercises will not likely be repeated.

Seniors in and out of the home should experience various interesting practices reinforcing the importance of easing into exercise. This should help your exercise experiences to become more positive and comfortable and promote long-term involvement in the strength training activities we will cover in the next chapter.

This chapter will guide you in doing warm-ups that are safe, effective, relevant, varied, and enjoyable. It will also help you build the necessary knowledge, understanding, and skills to exercise through the progressive stages.

Why You Need to Warm Up Your Body

Before you exercise, you've got to get your circulation going, raise the temperature in your muscles and tendons, and loosen them up. You must also release the fluid that lubricates your joints and gradually adjust your heart to match the rapid movements.

Your aerobic system takes a minute or two to kick in. In the meantime, nature has provided you with a backup plan—a fuel that burns without oxygen. You have just enough to carry you until your aerobic system kicks in. Only one rub: this anaerobic fuel loads your muscles with a waste product called lactic acid. And if you work too hard during these first two minutes and produce too much lactic acid, your muscles will cramp and ache.

Unless you enjoy pain and the possibility of a heart attack, starting slowly every time you exercise makes sense. You want all your body's systems operating at full power before turning on the steam. Otherwise, you'll feel like a boy who brought home a new exercise bike, hopped on it, pedaled furiously for about fifty seconds, then stopped. And that was it. He couldn't go on. Someone shoved a cactus down his throat when he wasn't looking and wrapped his legs in concrete blocks. He returned the bike to the store. Nothing was worth that kind of pain.

When you're in good shape and warm up gradually, you don't build enough lactic acid to notice its effects. But if you start at full tilt, as you may do in a race, or do a strenuous exercise where it's hard to start slowly, such as running or jumping rope, you may get winded. Your throat will feel dry, your muscles will become heavy, and you'll wonder how anyone could say exercising is fun. Lactic acid will accumulate in your body, and it will take two to fifteen minutes for your body to flush it away. Then, suddenly, you will breathe more easily, your throat will be moist again, your muscles will loosen up, and you will feel energized. At that point, your aerobic system will be working unencumbered. You've got your second wind. Yes, there is such a thing. It's a light, gentle relief and a sense of airiness.

Below are the specific benefits of doing warm-ups before engaging in any strength training activity:

- **It increases blood flow to your muscles:** Warming up increases blood flow to your muscles by dilating your blood vessels, which allows more blood to flow through them. When you engage in physical activity, your muscles need more oxygen and nutrients to sustain the effort. Warming up helps to increase the flow of blood to your muscles, which in turn helps to deliver more oxygen and nutrients to them. This can improve your muscle function and overall strength training performance.

- **It reduces the risk of injury:** There is an ongoing debate over the specific function and value of warm-ups and whether they decrease the risk of injury. The experimental evidence is likely to be partially conclusive, as it would be unethical for researchers to put subjects under conditions in which they may be injured. However, the combination of evidence from research findings and knowledge of muscle physiology, kinesiology, and exercise psychology supports the provision of a period of adjustment from rest to exercise as a prudent, protective measure for the body.

- **It improves your performance during your workout:** Warm-up also helps improve your performance by getting your muscles ready for the demands placed on them. When you engage in physical activity, your muscles need more oxygen and nutrients to sustain the effort. And as I have already explained, since warming up helps to increase blood flow to your muscles, they can help improve your muscle function and overall performance during your workout.

- **It improves the efficiency of movement:** Since warming up increases your heart rate and body temperature, it can help to improve your range of motion and make it easier for you to perform specific movements, which can, in turn, help to reduce the risk of muscle strains or pulls. Warming up helps your body achieve this goal by activating and priming the connections between your nerves and muscles. This can also help to reduce the risk of injury by allowing you to perform movements more efficiently and effectively. Finally, warming up can help to reduce muscle stiffness and increase blood flow to your muscles, which can help to reduce the risk of muscle cramps or other issues that can lead to injury.

A proper warm-up should include light cardiovascular activities to increase your heart rate and body temperature so you can take your joints through a full range of motion. What matters is that you start it slowly. It's much safer that way.

However, as you get into better shape, you may want to intensify your warm-up, and it's reassuring to know a second wind is waiting for you. If you're in excellent condition, you may get your second wind in a couple of minutes; however, if you're in poor condition, it may take ten or fifteen minutes.

Engage in Aerobic Activities

A warm-up for your strength training activity will take around ten to fifteen minutes. It involves light aerobic exercises appropriate for the activity you're about to perform.

Aerobic exercises that raise the heart rate and condition the heart and lungs are essential to health and fitness. I am often asked which aerobic exercise is best for fitness training and building aerobic strength. I always say that the best aerobic exercise is the one that you are most likely to do.

In most cases, this means doing whatever you will do for exercise—walking, running, cycling, and swimming—slowly and gently. So here we will look at how to get the most out of your aerobic exercise.

1. Walking

Walking is one of the best, and certainly one of the most versatile, ways to keep fit, and it is suitable for all fitness levels. It is a low-impact exercise that works the glutes, and leg muscles, particularly the quadriceps, and hamstrings.

Warm up by moving around at a leisurely pace for about five minutes to warm up your muscles. You can walk around your home (inside or out), but you will get just as much from a walk indoors on the treadmill, stationary bike, or even a rower when time is short, or the weather is poor.

Because it is easy to monitor and control how hard you work, walking is an excellent way to learn about how your heart rate responds to different exertion levels.

2. Walking up and down stairs (just a few at a time will do it)

Walking up and down stairs can be a great way to warm up and improve cardiovascular fitness. It is essential to use proper technique when walking up and down stairs to avoid injury.

Here are some tips for safe stair climbing:

- Take your time and go at a comfortable pace.

- Use the handrail if one is available, especially when going downstairs.

- Keep your feet straight ahead and your body centered over the stairs as you climb.

- Place your entire foot on each step rather than just the ball of your foot.

- Keep your eyes focused on the stairs before you rather than looking at your feet or the ground.

Following these tips can reduce your risk of falls and other injuries while climbing stairs.

3. Side-stepping

Side-stepping is an aerobic exercise that can help improve your endurance, coordination, and balance. You can increase your pace once you are in tune with your body and have the ability to go faster. You will need a flat surface and room to move to do side-stepping.

Here's how to get started:

- Stand with your feet spaced out and place your hands on your hips.

- Step to the left with your left foot, then step with your right foot to meet the other. Then, step to the right with your right foot and bring your left foot to meet your right foot. Continue alternating sides. You can increase your speed when you are able.

- As you side-step, keep your upper body upright and your feet pointed straight ahead.

- You can vary the speed and intensity of the exercise by increasing or decreasing the pace of your side steps.

- You can also add hand weights or a resistance band to increase the challenge of the exercise. Again, this is when you feel comfortable and able to perform this task.

Remember to warm up before starting any new exercise routine, and listen to your body to avoid overdoing it.

4. Swimming

Swimming is another fantastic warm-up exercise. It improves your fitness level and burns calories more effectively than many other forms of aerobic exercise. It also has a dual effect of building cardiovascular strength while toning and strengthening the body's major muscles.

A good program is essential to benefit from a swimming workout. Think of the swimming pool as an excellent source of low-impact activity and use swimming as the aerobic element of your training.

Focus on Your Breathing

Breathing is something you do all day and usually don't have to think about. However, paying attention to your breath cycles can be a powerful focus technique that can significantly add to the success of your warm-up routine.

Focusing on your breathing is essential during any physical activity, including warm-up exercises, as it will help you feel more alert. It can also help you maintain energy and focus and prevent fatigue and injuries. When warming up, focusing on deep, controlled breaths that fill your lungs and help oxygenate your muscles is important.

Here are the best practices for breathing during warm-up exercises:

- Take deep breaths through your nose and exhale through your mouth. This helps you get more oxygen into your body and can also help you relax.

- Try to maintain a steady rhythm of inhaling and exhaling as you exercise and help you maintain a consistent level of energy and focus.

- Focus on exhaling as you exert yourself, and inhale as you relax. For example, if you're running, exhale as you lift your feet off the ground and inhale as you land.

- Don't hold your breath. Keeping a consistent breathing pattern will help you maintain a steady flow of oxygen to your muscles and can also help reduce the risk of injury.

Remembering to breathe during a warm-up routine is the appropriate way to do it! Always remember to breathe in and out normally or comfortably rather than force a count of how long you should be breathing in and out. Many people tend to hold their breath, which can induce dizziness or lightheadedness and reduce the overall performance of their exercise.

When you first start, keep your exercise repetitions slow and controlled. As a result, assigning a specific count to how to breathe in and out makes no sense. For the best result, concentrate on managing your breathing and exhaling when exerting the maximum force.

Stay Hydrated

Staying hydrated is one of the most challenging factors to remember. Typically, drinking enough water is crucial for many reasons:

- It helps to regulate body temperature,

- It keeps joints well lubricated

- You can prevent infections by drinking more water

- It aids in the delivery of nutrients to cells

- Staying hydrated keeps your organs functioning properly.

Being well-hydrated also kick-starts your metabolism, promotes skin health, and improves sleep quality, cognition, and mood.

More importantly, staying hydrated during any physical activity, including warm-up exercises, can help you maintain your energy levels, improve your performance, and reduce the risk of injury. Here are the best practices for staying hydrated during warm-up exercises:

- Drink water before, during, and after your warm-up. Aim to drink at least eight ounces of water before exercising, and continue to drink small sips throughout your warm-up.

- Keep a water bottle with you during your warm-up. This makes it easy for you to stay hydrated and help prevent dehydration.

- Listen to your body's thirst signals. If you're feeling thirsty, it's a sign that you need to drink more water.

- Avoid sugary or caffeinated drinks during your warm-up. These drinks can dehydrate your body and interfere with your performance.

Remember, staying hydrated is vital for maintaining energy levels and helping your body perform at its best. So be sure to drink plenty of water before, during, and after your warm-up exercises.

According to experts, the average woman should drink eleven cups of water daily, while men should drink sixteen cups. (A good rule of thumb is to drink 1/3 of your body weight.) Not all of those cups must contain ordinary water; you can flavor with fruit or vegetables (lemons, berries, orange, or cucumber slices) or coffee or tea. However, as previously said, it is better to avoid sugar-sweetened beverages when trying to stay hydrated.

Limited time is often an excuse for not paying enough attention to warm-ups. However, if you view a warm-up more as a lead-in activity than a separate, tagged-on section, it is far more likely to be relevant, integral, and valued. It would be best if you established good habits in terms of warming up early on, and it should become an accepted element of every exercise session we will cover starting from Chapter 4 through Chapter 6.

It's important to remember that the goal of a warm-up is not to tire yourself out but to gently prepare your body for the physical activity that is to come, so don't push yourself too hard. Aim for about five to ten minutes of warm-up exercises before you start your workout. And if you're feeling tired or out of breath, take a break and walk for a few minutes before continuing your warm-up.

Key Takeaways

- A warm-up is a group of exercises performed just before an activity, which helps the body to adjust from a state of rest to exercise.

- Easing into strength training exercises ensures that the activity experience is more comfortable and that there is less likelihood of injury.

- A warm-up will take around ten to fifteen minutes and involves light aerobic activities like walking, marching, and swimming.

- Paying attention to your breathing can be a powerful focus technique that can significantly add to the success of your warm-up routine.

- Staying hydrated during any physical activity, including warm-up exercises, can help you maintain your energy levels, improve your performance, and reduce the risk of injury.

Chapter 4: The First Three Weeks of Your Journey

"Aging is not lost youth but a new stage of opportunity and strength."

– Betty Friedan

This chapter will discuss the four basic exercises you should focus on during the first three weeks of your strength training journey. As we age, our bodies undergo natural changes that affect our ability to move and perform everyday activities. However, these basic exercises can help seniors maintain independence, improve their health, and prevent chronic diseases.

Before we proceed, you must understand the importance of starting slowly. Starting slowly and gradually increasing the workouts' intensity is crucial for seniors, as it allows them to safely and effectively build up their strength, endurance, and overall fitness. It can also help them ease into their workout routine and avoid injury, burnout, and a lack of motivation to continue exercising.

For example, if you are new to push-ups, start by doing two sets of ten reps and gradually increase the time you spend doing push-ups over a few weeks.

Gradually increasing the intensity of your workouts will also help you maintain your motivation. When you see the benefits of your exercise program, such as improved stamina and strength, you are more likely to continue exercising. Additionally, starting slowly and gradually increasing the intensity of workouts can help you avoid burnout, which can happen when you push yourself to exceed set limits too soon.

It is also important to listen to your body and not push yourself too hard. Refrain from ego-lifting or thinking that you can do it all. You should stop and rest If you feel pain or discomfort during a workout. You should also consult with your doctor before starting this exercise program to ensure it is safe. Now that we've gotten that out of the way, it's time to get started on the four basic exercises.

Reach for the Stars

"Reach for the Stars" is a simple exercise involving "walking" on a wall with your arms and fingers. This activity has been shown to have cognitive benefits, as it can help to improve fine motor skills, coordination, and attention.

This exercise also has several benefits for seniors, including the following:

- **Improved dexterity:** The exercise helps to strengthen the movement and control of your fingers and grip; it also increases the flexibility of your arms, back, and shoulders. In addition, it is a great way to keep the fingers nimble, making it easier for you to perform daily tasks such as writing, typing, and buttoning clothes.

- **Increased hand strength:** The "Reach for the Stars" exercise also helps to strengthen the muscles in your hands and fingers, which can help to prevent injuries and improve overall hand function.

- **Reduced risk of Arthritis:** Regular hand and finger exercises can also help to reduce the risk of developing conditions such as arthritis, as they keep the joints mobile and prevent stiffness.

- **Improved overall hand health:** Finger matching exercises can also help to improve blood circulation and reduce the risk of hand injuries by keeping the fingers flexible and strong.

Here are the steps to practice the "Reach for the Stars" exercise:

- Sit in a comfortable, armless chair with your feet flat on the floor, shoulder-width apart.

- As you are seated, hold your hands in front of you, with your palms against an imaginary wall.

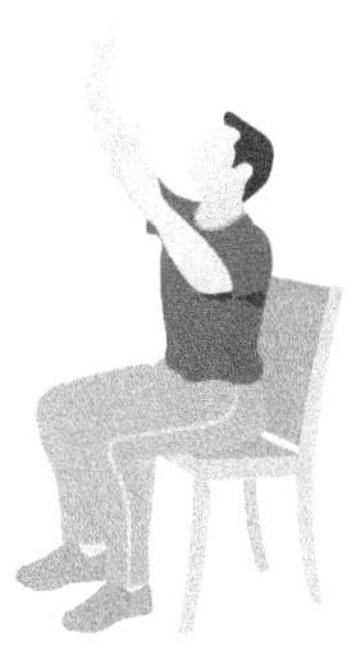

Slowly use your fingers to climb the imaginary wall before you until your arms are above your head. Once you reach the top, wiggle your fingers for about ten seconds before walking them back down. Perform the "Reach for the Stars" exercise for two sets of ten reps; in other words, ten repetitions twice. (If you cannot do ten reps, do as many as possible.)

- Next, try to reach your arms behind your back while sitting or standing shoulder-width apart. If you can, reach for the opposite elbow with each hand or get as close to the elbow as you can. Then hold that position for eight to ten seconds and release when you start feeling a stretch in your back, arms, and chest.

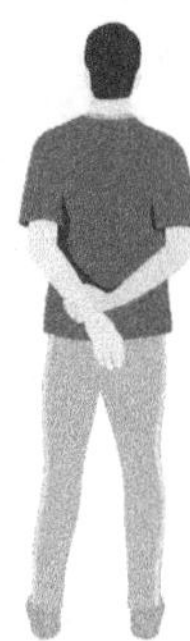

- Finally, clasp your hands together while standing or sitting and then push them out, facing away from you. Stretch forth your arms so that they are parallel to the ground, palms toward the imaginary wall. Next, straighten your back and shoulders, then curl them forward. You should feel a stretch in your wrist and upper back. Hold the position for eight to ten seconds. You can also perform this exercise while seated.

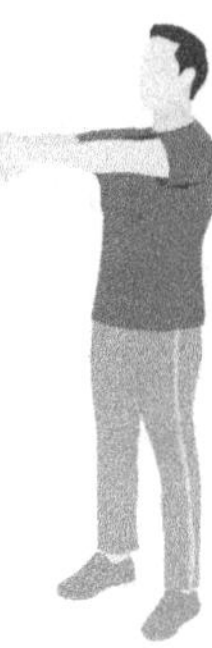

If you want to add a different exercise, you can do these variations of the "Reach for the Stars":

- **Finger tapping:** You can practice this variation by placing your hand flat on a table and tapping each finger on the table, one at a time, starting with the thumb and working your way down to the pinky finger.

- **Finger curl:** You can practice finger curling by holding a small object, such as a pencil or pen, in your hand and making a fist around it, squeezing it tightly. Then release the squeeze and repeat several times.

- **Finger extension:** You can do this variation by holding your hand out in front of you, palm down, and spreading your fingers as wide as you can. Then bring them back together and repeat several times.

- **Hand squeeze:** You can do this variation by squeezing a rubber ball or another hand gripper to strengthen your hand and fingers.

- **Fingerpicking:** You can practice this variation by holding small objects, like coins or marbles, and picking them up one by one with different fingers, starting with your thumb and working your way down to your pinky.

- **Key turning:** You can do this variation by holding a key and turning it back and forth with different fingers, starting with your thumb and working your way down to your pinky.

- **Pinch and spread:** In this variation, you can hold a small object, such as a pencil or pen, and close your fist around it. Next, you could spread your fingers apart and close them again.

It's important to keep the pace slow and steady to avoid sudden movements that could cause injury. As you get comfortable with the exercise, you can increase the speed and do more sets.

Heel Lift/Standing on Your Toes

The heel lift exercise, also known as "Standing on Your Toes," is a simple but effective exercise that can help you improve the strength and flexibility of your calf, ankle, and foot muscles. This exercise has several benefits, including the following:

- **Improved balance and stability:** Heel lifts can help you to improve your balance and stability, as it strengthens the muscles in the calf and ankle, which can help to alleviate joint pain, especially in the knees, and reduce the risk of falls in older adults.

- **Increased muscle strength:** Heel lifts target the muscles in the calf, which are responsible for lifting the heel off the ground. Regular exercise can help increase muscle strength and improve overall leg function.

- **Reduced risk of injury:** Strong calf muscles can help to prevent common injuries, such as strains and sprains, by providing better support to the ankle and foot.

- **Improved posture:** Heel lifts can also help to improve your posture since it strengthens the muscles in your calf, which can help to align the spine and reduce the risk of lower back pain. The exercise opens your hips and strengthens your core and feet.

- **Improved athletic performance:** Athletes often use heel lifts to enhance their performance, as they help to increase power and explosiveness in the lower leg, which can help to improve their running and jumping ability.

Here are the steps for the heel lift exercise:

- Stand behind a sturdy chair with your feet shoulder-width apart and place your arms by your sides. It would be best not to lean on the chair; it is there to help if needed.

- Slowly raise your heels as high as you can while maintaining your balance.

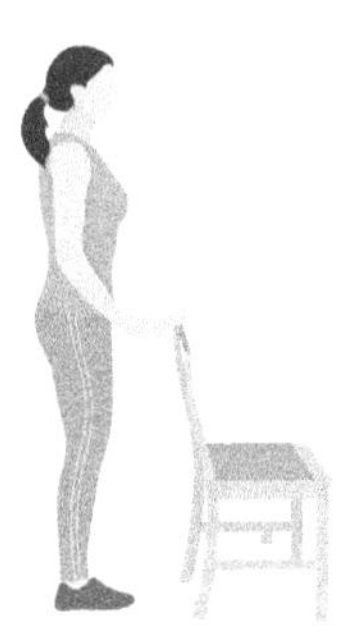

Stay in the position for three to five seconds before slowly lowering your heels back to the ground.

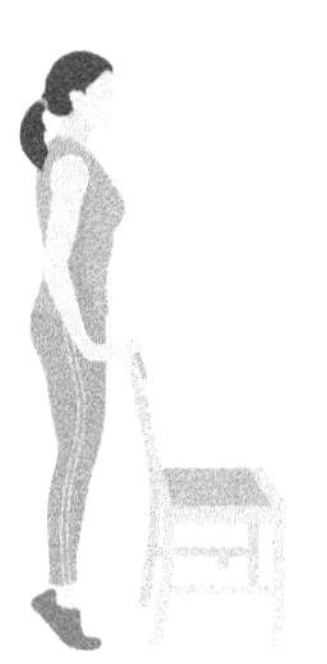

Do the heel lift exercise for ten repetitions, take a short break, and then do another ten repetitions, working both legs. Again, I will stress if you cannot do this many at first, do what is possible.

If you want, you can do these variations of the heel lift exercise:

Seated heel lifts: Sit on a bench or chair with your feet on the floor, and your knees bent to perform this variant. Then, raise your heels slowly off the floor, hold them for a moment, and lower them back down.

- **Toe lifts:** To perform this variation, stand with your feet shoulder-width apart and place your arms by your sides. Then, raise your toes as high as possible while maintaining your balance. Hold the stance for a few seconds before slowly lowering your toes.

- **Step-up heel lift:** This variation can be done by standing in front of a step or bench. Step up with one foot, raise your heel as high as possible, hold that position for a moment, and lower your heel back down.

It's important to note that you should use a level surface to perform the exercise, like the floors of a gym. And as you become more comfortable with the exercise, you can increase the number of repetitions and try to perform the activity on one leg at a time.

Additionally, if you have any joint pain or arthritis, you should consult your doctor before starting any exercise.

Wall Push-Ups

Wall push-ups are a modified version of the traditional push-up exercise that can help improve your upper body strength and endurance. This exercise offers seniors several benefits, including the following:

- **Improved upper body strength:** Wall push-ups can help to improve upper body strength by working the chest, shoulders, and arms. This can help seniors to perform daily activities such as lifting groceries or reaching for objects on high shelves easily.

- **Increased endurance:** Wall push-ups can also help to increase endurance by working the large muscle groups of the upper body, which can help seniors perform more exercise repetitions, leading to greater overall fitness.

- **Improved posture:** Wall push-ups can help to improve posture by working the muscles of the chest and shoulders, which can help to align the spine and reduce the risk of lower back pain.

- **Reduced risk of injury:** Strong upper body muscles can help to prevent common injuries, such as strains and sprains, by providing better support to the shoulder and arm.

- **Improved bone density:** Weight-bearing exercises, like wall push-ups, have been shown to impact bone density, particularly in the upper body, positively.

Here are the steps for the wall push-up exercise:

- Stand facing a wall with your feet apart and your hands placed on the wall at shoulder height. Your hands should be slightly wider than shoulder-width apart and slightly below shoulder level.

- Slowly bend your elbows and lower your head toward the wall, keeping your body straight. Your whole body should move forward, hinging at the ankles. But whatever you do, your feet should not move.

- Once your elbows reach a ninety-degree angle, push back up to the starting position.

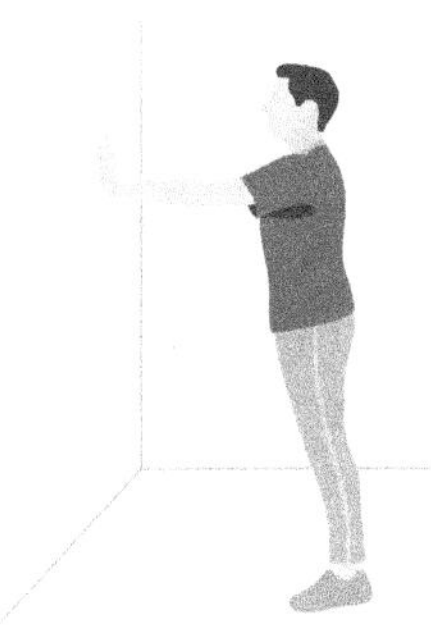

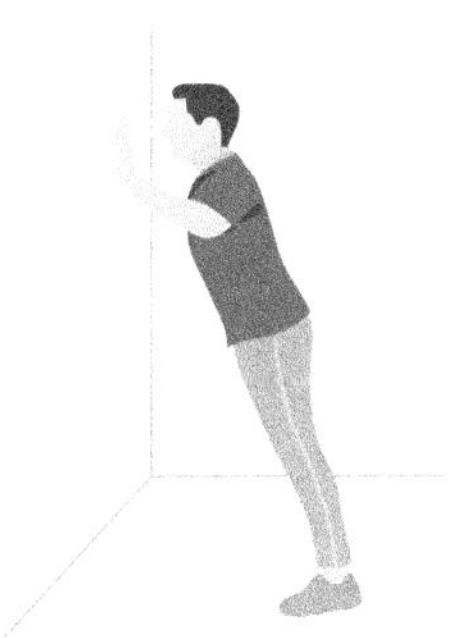

It would help if you did wall push-ups for ten repetitions, take a short break, and add another ten repetitions. That is, you should do two sets of ten reps. But if you find ten reps too hard, start with a smaller amount; make sure you are targeting your arms, chest, back, and shoulders.

If you want, you can do these more challenging variations of the wall push-ups exercise:

- **Incline wall push-ups:** You can perform this variation by placing your hands higher on the wall, making the exercise easier.

- **Decline wall push-ups:** You can perform this variation by placing your feet further away, making the exercise more challenging.

- **Single-arm wall push-ups:** You can practice this variation by performing the push-up exercise one arm at a time.

- **Countertop push-ups:** This is a variation of the same exercise, but instead of pressing against a wall, you push against the edge of a countertop. You will need to move your feet backward after placing your hands on the tabletop, again a little wider than shoulder-width apart.

The difficulty of these workouts is primarily determined by how far you go. Lowering your head or chest to the wall or countertop will be much more challenging if you merely lower it a few inches. So, when needed, alter your range of motion.

You can try each push-up variation and select the one that works best for you. By incorporating wall push-ups into your strength training routine, you can help to improve the strength and endurance of the upper body muscles, which can help to improve overall upper body function and reduce the risk of injury.

Stand Up/Sit Down (Pop Squats)

Pop squats are a chair activity and an excellent exercise for seniors, which you can do to improve the strength and flexibility of the muscles in your legs, hips, and glutes. But you do not have to be a senior to benefit from the squat pop exercise. For example, you must build up your strength if recovering from an accident or illness. The squat pop exercise is a great way to achieve that goal.

You do this exercise by performing a squat while sitting on the edge of a chair, using the chair as a guide for proper form. Here are the benefits of pop squats:

- **Improved leg strength:** Pop squats target the muscles in the legs, including the quadriceps, hamstrings, and glutes. Regularly performing this exercise can help increase muscle strength, improve overall leg function, and reduce the risk of falls.

- **Improved balance and stability:** This exercise also helps to improve balance and stability by strengthening the muscles in the legs and hips, which can help to reduce the risk of falls in older adults.

- **Reduced risk of injury:** Strong leg muscles can help to prevent common injuries, such as strains and sprains, by providing better support to the knee and ankle.

- **Improved flexibility:** Pop squats are a low-impact exercise, making them easy on the joints and an excellent option for seniors or those recovering from an injury.

- **Convenience:** You can do this exercise anywhere, as long as there's a chair nearby.

- **Bodyweight exercise:** Pop squats are a bodyweight exercise, which means you don't need any equipment.

Outlined below are the steps for the pop squat exercise:

- Start by standing in front of a sturdy chair, with your feet spaced out and your hands on your knees.

- Now, bend your knees and pretend you are going to sit as you try to keep your weight on your heels.

- Then pause and stand up, using your legs to push yourself up.

- Slowly lower yourself back down to the chair, keeping your back straight and your weight in your heels.

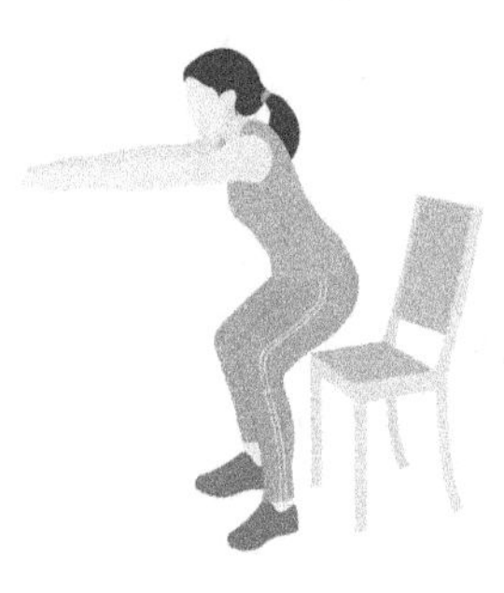

(If you cannot keep your arms forward, use your arms to steady yourself on the sides of the chair.)

You should do the pop squat exercise for ten repetitions, take a short break, and do another ten repetitions. (I found this exercise was hard on my lower back with my injury. I started doing just one at a time. Please do what you are able. I can now do these with no pain or struggle.)

If you want, you can do these more challenging variations of the pop squat activity:

- **Single-leg chair squats:** You can practice this variation by performing the squat movement with one leg at a time, which can help to increase balance and stability.

- **Pulse squats:** You can practice this variation by performing a series of small squats instead of one full squat. This can help to increase muscle endurance and burn more calories.

- **Chair squats with weights:** You can practice this variation by holding a lightweight, such as a dumbbell or a water bottle while performing the squat. This can help to increase muscle strength and burn more calories.

- **Chair squats with a resistance band:** You can practice this variation by attaching a resistance band around your legs, above the knee, and performing the squat movement. The bonus of this exercise is it can increase muscle strength and burn more calories.

- **Isometric chair squats:** You can practice this variation by performing a squat movement and holding the position at the bottom of the squat for a few seconds. This can help to increase muscle endurance and burn more calories.

- **Chair jump squats:** You can practice this variation by squatting and jumping off the chair. The benefit is to help increase cardiovascular endurance and burn more calories. This exercise should be used when you are confident in your ability and training.

But if you find the exercise too hard, you can use your hands for support or put your hands on your knees to help push yourself up. If the movement is still too hard, have someone assist you by standing in front of you so you can grab their hands and pull yourself up. Then, gradually, you can reduce the amount of help you need.

The squat pop exercise targets your upper thighs, buttock muscles, and the bones in your hips and spine. So, keep your back straight and your abs tight during each lift. This supports the spine, prevents injury, and targets the correct muscles.

According to research, performing these four basic strengthening exercises in the first three weeks of your strength training is safe and beneficial for men and women of all ages, including those in poor health. People with health issues, such as heart disease or arthritis, may benefit most from an exercise regimen that includes weight lifting a few times weekly.

Strength training activities, especially with regular cardiovascular exercises, can significantly impact your mental and emotional health. Meanwhile, in the following chapter, we'll look at four more exercises to add to your strength training program.

Key Takeaways

- Starting slowly and gradually increasing the intensity of your workouts is crucial, as it allows you to safely and effectively build up your strength, endurance, and overall fitness.

- It is important to listen to your body and not push yourself too hard. Refrain from ego-lifting or thinking that you can do it all. **You should stop and rest if you feel pain or discomfort during a workout.**

- "Reach for the Stars" is a simple exercise with cognitive benefits, as it can help to improve fine motor skills, coordination, and attention.

- The heel lift exercise helps you improve the strength and flexibility of your calf, ankle, and foot muscles.

- Wall push-ups can help to increase endurance by working the large muscle groups of the upper body. This can help seniors perform more exercise repetitions, increasing overall fitness.

- Pop squats help to improve balance and stability by strengthening the muscles in the legs and hips, which can help to reduce the risk of falls in older adults.

Chapter 5: The Next Four Exercises to Add to Your Routine

"It does not matter how slowly you go as long as you do not stop."

– Confucius

As you progress in your exercise routine and become more comfortable with your current workout, you want to gradually increase the intensity by doing more exercises. And that's what we will do in this chapter; we will discuss four new exercises to add to your strength training routine.

Incorporating these new exercises will help to target different muscle groups that can help to improve your overall fitness and prevent muscle imbalances. You will also have the freedom to vary the intensity of your workout to avoid boredom, improve your overall wellness, and keep your body challenged.

So, why not try these new exercises or switch up the order of exercises to keep your body guessing? The most important thing is to be consistent with your exercise routine, stick to it, and make it a part of your daily routine.

Again, it's important to note that you should always consult your doctor before increasing your workout's intensity. Also, listen to your body and not push yourself too hard. As I already explained, a gradual increase in intensity and proper form is the key to avoiding injury and burnout.

Step Climb (Moving up in the World)

Step climb, also known as step-up, allows seniors to improve their strength and endurance in their legs, hips, and glutes. This exercise can use a step or bench, and it's a great way to improve balance and stability, reducing the risk of falls in older adults. Here are some of the benefits of step-up exercises for seniors:

- **Improved leg strength:** Step climbs exercise targets the muscles in the legs, including the quadriceps, hamstrings, and glutes, which can help to increase muscle strength and improve overall leg function.

- **Improved balance and stability:** It also helps to improve balance and stability by strengthening the muscles in the legs and hips, which can help to reduce the risk of falls in older adults.

- **Reduced risk of injury:** Strong leg muscles can help to prevent common injuries, such as strains and sprains, by providing better support to the knees and ankles.

- **Improved cardiovascular fitness:** The step-up exercise can also help to improve cardiovascular fitness by increasing the heart rate, which can help to improve overall health.

- **Low impact:** Step up is a low-impact exercise, making it easy on the joints and an excellent option for seniors or those recovering from an injury.

- **Convenience:** The exercise can be done anywhere, as long as a step or a bench is nearby.

- **Versatility:** Step-ups can be adjusted to match the senior's ability and fitness level by using different height steps or adding weights.

Outlined below are the steps for the step-up exercise:

- Start by standing before a step with your feet spaced out and your hands on your hips. Make sure your feet are flat on the floor and you have a rail to hold onto.

- Step up onto the step with your left foot, then lift your right foot to meet it as if you want to climb the stairs.

- Now, step back down with your right foot only, and then bring your left foot down to meet it.

- Use a five-count method to go up and down.

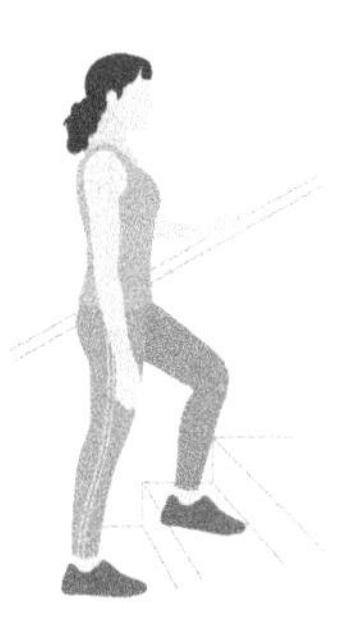

You should do the step climb exercise for ten repetitions, take a short break, and do another ten repetitions or, two sets of ten reps.

Always do what you are capable of. Build your endurance at your pace.

Several variations of the step climb exercise can be done to target different muscle groups and increase the difficulty of the exercise. Some examples include the following:

- **Reverse step climbs:** Step back onto a box or bench. More emphasis is on the glutes and hamstrings.

- **Lateral step climbs:** Step up and across a box or bench rather than straight up. This targets the adductors (inner thigh muscles) more heavily.

- **Single-leg step climbs:** Perform the exercise on one leg at a time rather than two. This increases the balance and stability challenge and heavily targets the glutes, quads, and core.

- **Weighted step climbs:** Hold dumbbells or a barbell while performing the exercise. The resistance makes the exercise more challenging.

Start with low repetitions as you switch your feet and repeat the process. Also, it's always best to start with your body weight and progress to adding leg weights or increasing your step height. However, consult a personal trainer or doctor before increasing your workouts' intensity.

Bicep Curl (Strong Like Bull)

A bicep curl is an exercise that primarily targets the bicep muscles. You can perform this exercise using your lightest equipment, such as dumbbells, barbells, or resistance bands. Using weights will help to boost your grip strength for healthier hands.

Here are some of the benefits of performing bicep curls regularly:

- **Increased muscle mass:** Bicep curls can help increase the size and strength of the biceps, improving upper body appearance and strength.

- **Improved arm definition:** Bicep curls can also help define and shape the biceps, giving the arms a more toned and sculpted appearance.

- **Improved grip strength:** Bicep curls require gripping two weights, which can help improve grip strength and the ability to perform activities that require a firm grip.

- **Better functional strength:** Bicep curls work the muscles in your upper arms that improve functional strength and help bend your elbows, which you need for activities such as carrying groceries, lifting children, pulling the door, and performing tasks that require upper body strength.

- **Increased bone density:** Bicep curls, like any other weight training exercise, can help increase bone density, lowering the risk of osteoporosis.

- **Improved posture:** Strong biceps can help improve posture by keeping the shoulders back and chest out, making you look taller and more confident.

Here is a basic description of how to perform a bicep curl using dumbbells:

- Stand or sit with your feet spaced out and hold a dumbbell in both hands with an underhand grip.

- Keep your elbows close to your sides and your palms facing up.

- Lift dumbbells by curling your arms (bending your elbows) to your shoulders, with your palms facing your body while keeping your upper arms stationary.

- Squeeze your biceps and hold at the apex of the exercise.

- Return the dumbbells to the starting position with control.

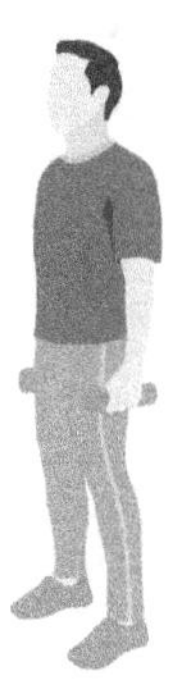

Do the bicep curls for ten repetitions (five going up and five going down), take a short break, and then do another ten repetitions. That is two sets of ten reps.

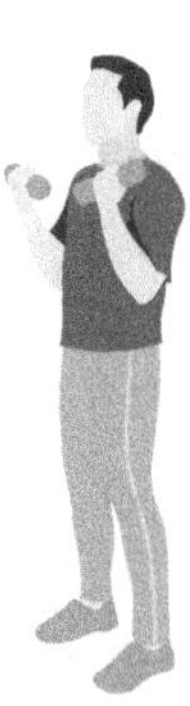

If you want, you can do these more challenging variations of the bicep curls exercise:

Hammer curls: Instead of holding the weights with your palms facing forward, hold them facing each other. This variation targets the brachioradialis muscle on the top of the forearm and the biceps.

- **Incline dumbbell curls:** Instead of standing upright, perform the exercise while lying on an incline bench. This variation places more emphasis on the long head of the biceps muscle.

- **Concentration curls:** Sit on a bench or chair, place your elbow on the inside of your thigh, hold the weights, and curl them toward your shoulder; this isolation movement explicitly targets the bicep muscle.

- **Preacher curls:** Sit on a preacher bench, hold a barbell with an underhand grip, and curl the weight toward your shoulders; this variation also isolates the biceps.

- **21's curls:** This technique is where you perform seven curls from the bottom of the rep, seven curls from the middle, and seven curls from the top, giving your biceps a good burn.

Above all, it is vital to use proper form and not swing the weight or use momentum to lift it; this will help you target the muscle effectively and avoid any injury.

Overhead Press

The overhead press, also known as the military press, is a strength training exercise that targets the back, shoulders, triceps, and upper chest. The exercise uses a barbell or a pair of dumbbells. The basic movement involves lifting the weight overhead while standing or sitting, starting with the weight at the shoulders and extending the arms overhead. The best part is that you can customize the exercise to suit your fitness level as you get stronger.

Here are the several benefits the overhead press offers:

- **Increased upper body strength:** The overhead press can help seniors build upper body strength, improving their ability to perform daily activities and reducing the risk of falls.

- **Improved posture:** It can also help seniors improve their posture by strengthening the shoulders and upper chest. This can help reduce back pain risk and improve their overall appearance.

- **Increased bone density:** Weight-bearing exercises like the overhead press can help increase bone density, lowering the risk of osteoporosis and fractures.

- **Improved cardiovascular health:** The overhead press is a weight-bearing exercise that can be cardio-intensive, which can help to improve cardiovascular health and increase overall fitness levels.

- **Improved coordination:** The overhead press requires coordination and balance, which can help to improve overall coordination and balance.

- **Increased self-esteem:** Regular exercise can help seniors feel better physically, leading to increased self-esteem and a better overall quality of life.

Here are the basic steps for performing the overhead press exercise:

- Begin by standing or sitting with your feet shoulder-width apart and your core engaged.

- Hold a pair of dumbbells or a barbell at shoulder level with your palms facing out.

- Slowly press the weights overhead to a count of three, keeping your elbows close to your body and your core engaged.

- As you press the weights overhead, exhale and extend your arms fully

- To a count of three, slowly lower the weights back to the starting position, inhaling as you do so.

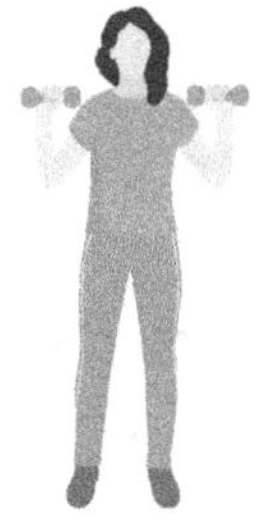

Do the overhead press exercise for ten repetitions, take a short break, and do another ten repetitions. That is two sets of ten reps.

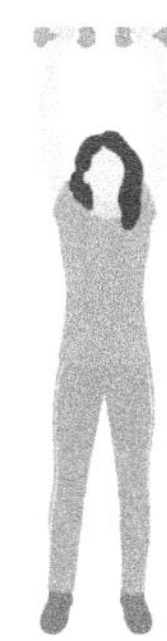

There are several variations of the overheard press exercise as well:

Seated overhead press: You can perform this variation while sitting on a bench; this can help to stabilize the upper body and reduce the risk of falling.

Standing overhead barbell press: You can perform this variation with a barbell while standing; this can be more challenging as the core muscles are engaged more.

- **Standing dumbbell overhead press:** You can perform this variation with a pair of dumbbells while standing; this variation can help to improve balance and symmetry.

- **Push press:** This variation combines a squat and an overhead press and can help increase power and explosiveness.

- **Arnold press:** This exercise is a variation of the dumbbell press; however, it targets the shoulders from a different angle and involves the rotation of the shoulders.

- **Z-press:** You can perform this variation sitting on the ground with your legs straight; this exercise can help to increase core stability and engage the legs.

However, seniors need to take a few precautions when performing this exercise:

- **Start with lighter weights:** Seniors should begin with lesser weights and gradually raise the weight as their strength increases and they grow more comfortable with the exercise.

- **Focus on good form:** Proper form is crucial when performing the overhead press. The senior should keep the core engaged, the back straight, and the shoulders back.

- **Avoid locking out the elbow:** Locking out the elbow can put excessive stress on the joint and increase the risk of injury.

- **Use a seated position:** Performing the overhead press while sitting can help to stabilize the upper body and reduce the risk of falling.

- **Warm-up is important:** Seniors must warm up before performing the overhead press. They could do light cardio and shoulder rotations to help prepare the body for the exercise.

In addition, it's important to remember that every senior is different and may have different physical limitations, so it's essential to check with your doctor or physical therapist before starting any new workout.

Side Hip Raise

The side hip raise exercise, known as the side plank leg lift, targets the glutes, hips, and core muscles. This exercise can help to improve stability, balance, and strength in these areas.

Here are some of the benefits of performing side hip raises for seniors:

- **Improved balance and stability:** The side hip raise requires balance and stability, which can help with a better range of motion in the hips, improve overall balance, and reduce the risk of falls.

- **Increased core strength:** This exercise also targets the core muscles, which can help to improve core strength and stability, which can help to improve your posture and eliminate the risk of you having back pain.

- **Increased hip strength:** The side hip raise targets the hip muscles, which can help to improve hip strength and stability, and overall mobility.

- **Reduced risk of injury:** Strong glutes and muscles can help avoid damage, as they support the lower back and hips.

- **Improved bone density:** Weight-bearing exercises like the side hip raise can help increase bone density, lowering the risk of osteoporosis and fractures.

- **Improved functional strength:** The side hip raise can help to improve functional strength, which can help seniors perform daily activities more efficiently, such as climbing stairs or standing up from a seat.

Here is a basic description of how to perform the side hip raise exercise:

- Start in a side plank position, with your feet, elbow, and forearm on a firm surface, like the sofa or the floor.

- Keep your hips lifted and your body straight from your head to your feet. Also, make sure not to lock your knees.

- Slowly raise your top leg as high as possible without letting your hips drop.

- Hold a moment, then lower your leg back down.

Perform this exercise for ten repetitions for one side of your hips, then repeat the activity on the other side. That should equal two sets of ten reps.

Here are a few variations of the side hip raise
exercise that can provide a more challenging
workout and target the muscle groups in
different ways:

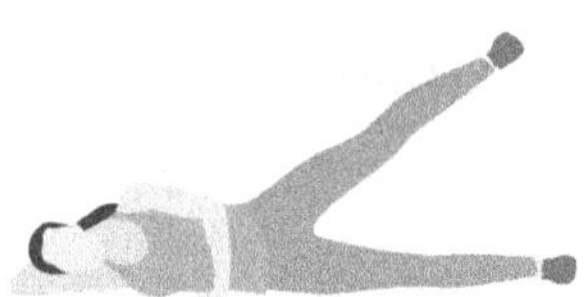

- **Elevated side hip raises:** Perform
  the exercise with your feet on an
  elevated surface, such as a bench
  or step. This variation increases the
  range of motion and makes the
  exercise more challenging.

- **Side hip raise with a resistance band:** Place a resistance band
  around your legs, just above the knee, and perform the exercise;
  this variation will increase the resistance on your hip muscles.

- **Weighted side hip raises:** Hold a dumbbell or weight plate with
  your top hand during the exercise. This variation increases the
  resistance and makes the exercise more challenging.

- **Reverse side hip raise:** Perform the exercise with your feet facing
  forward instead of facing backward. This variation targets the
  glutes and hip flexors differently.

- **Single leg side hip raises:** Perform the exercise on one leg at a
  time; this increases the balance and stability challenge and targets
  the glutes, quads, and core more heavily.

- **Side hip raise with a knee raise:** Instead of lifting your leg
  straight, lift your knee to your chest; this variation targets the
  oblique muscles more heavily.

I recommend you start the side hip raise with your body weight and
progress to added weight as you get comfortable and stronger with the
program. Also, keep your core engaged and your body in a straight line
throughout the exercise; it's also important not to let your hips sag or
rotate during the movement. Finally, keep your breathing steady and
controlled throughout the training.

These four additional strength training exercises we covered in this chapter will benefit you long-term as they will help improve muscle mass, strength, overall health, and overall functional ability and reduce your risk of falling.

These activities can also help increase bone density, lowering the risk of osteoporosis and fractures. You will also have a low risk of chronic diseases such as obesity, diabetes, heart disease, and high blood pressure. Additionally, strength training increases metabolism, aiding in weight loss and maintaining a healthy weight.

Ultimately, you will enjoy an improved mood, eliminate symptoms of depression and anxiety, and improve your overall quality of life. We will take our strength training journey a step further in the next chapter, as I will introduce you to the final four strength training exercises to add to your routine.

Key Takeaways

- Incorporating new exercises into your workout routine will help to target different muscle groups that can help to improve overall fitness and prevent muscle imbalances.

- The step climb exercise targets the muscles in the legs, including the quadriceps, hamstrings, and glutes, which can help to increase muscle strength and improve overall leg function.

- Bicep curls work the muscles in your upper arms that improve functional strength, which you need for activities such as carrying groceries, lifting children, pulling the door, and performing tasks that require upper body strength.

- The overhead press is a weight-bearing exercise that can be cardio-intensive, which can help to improve cardiovascular health and increase overall fitness levels.

- The side hip raise can help to improve functional strength, which can help seniors perform daily activities more efficiently, such as climbing stairs or standing up from a seat.

- Always stop if you experience any discomfort.

- Only do what you are capable of doing. You can always increase your reps as you continue on your journey.

- The most important thing is to be consistent with your exercise routine, stick to it, and make it a part of your daily rou

Chapter 6: The Final Four Exercises to Complete Your Routine

"*Pain is temporary. Quitting lasts forever.*"

– Lance Armstrong

This chapter will introduce you to the final four exercises to complete your strength training routine. But this time, we will focus more on working your lower body. Combining the four exercises in this chapter with the previous eight will do wonders for your physical and mental health.

Now, exercising the lower body is important for several reasons. The lower body includes the muscles of the hips, legs, and feet, which are the body's foundation and support and move the rest of the body. Strong legs and hips help maintain balance, stability, and good posture, which are crucial for preventing injuries and maintaining good overall health.

One of the main benefits of exercising the lower body is that it can help improve cardiovascular health. The muscles of the lower body are significant, and working them can help boost metabolism, which helps burn more calories and promote weight loss. Additionally, regular exercise of the lower body can decrease your risk of chronic diseases such as diabetes, heart disease, and cancer.

Another benefit of exercising the lower body is improving overall physical function. Many daily activities, such as walking, carrying little children, climbing stairs, and standing, require using the lower body muscles. And strong leg muscles will make these activities more manageable and less tiring, which can help us maintain independence as we age.

In addition to the physical benefits, exercising the lower body can positively affect mental well-being. Regular exercise improves mood, reduces stress and anxiety, and promotes overall mental health.

Finally, strong lower body muscles can also help improve your aerobic exercise performance, especially in running, swimming, and any activity involving quick direction changes. Working your lower body muscles can also boost your performance in soccer, basketball, and track events, as these sports rely heavily on the strength and power of your lower body muscles.

However, while several exercises aim to strengthen lower body muscles, we will focus on only the four major ones that are proven to impact all the vital areas of the lower body and are essential for overall fitness and well-being.

Hamstring Curl (Give Yourself a Kick!)

The hamstring curl, also known as leg curl, is a popular exercise that targets the muscles in the back of the thigh, known as the hamstrings. The hamstrings are a group of three muscles (the biceps femoris, semitendinosus, and semimembranosus) that run from the hip to the knee and are responsible for knee flexion and hip extension.

The hamstring curl is an effective exercise for seniors that helps to develop strength and power in the hamstrings. Below are some of the benefits of doing the hamstring curl:

- **Improved muscle tone and definition:** Hamstring curls help tone and strengthen the muscles in the back of the thigh, making the lower body more defined and attractive.

- **Increased lower body strength:** The hamstrings are a vital muscle group for overall lower body strength and stability. So, strong hamstrings can improve your performance in sports and other physical activities and help prevent injury.

- **Enhanced athletic performance:** Hamstring curls can help to improve your running, jumping, and reflexes, making them an essential exercise for athletes and sports enthusiasts.

- **Reduced risk of injury:** Weak hamstrings usually cause knee and lower back injuries. So, by strengthening the hamstrings, you can reduce your risk of injury and improve your overall mobility and stability.

- **Balanced muscle development:** The hamstrings are often overlooked in many workout routines, but doing hamstring curls helps to maintain balance and symmetry in the legs. When your hamstrings become stronger, it can lead to better posture, walking, and running.

- **Improved core:** Hamstring curls also engage and strengthen the core muscles and glutes.

- **Versatility:** Hamstring curls have many variations, both machine-based and bodyweight exercises, which you can do to strengthen your hamstrings. This can help you target different fitness levels and goals depending on which variation you choose.

To perform the hamstring curl, follow these steps:

- Begin by standing behind a sturdy chair with your upper body straight. It would be best if you did not allow your body to swing.

- Also, keep your legs in place and try not to move your hips.

- Curl your leg slowly toward your glutes while keeping your knees straight down.

- Hold that position for a while, then slowly lower your leg to the starting position.

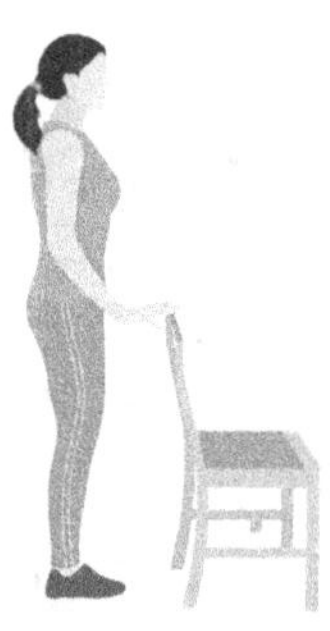

It would help if you did the hamstring curl exercise for ten repetitions, take a short break, and then do another ten repetitions for the other leg—two sets of ten reps for both legs.

Only lift as high as is comfortable. You will improve as you continue your journey.

- The most common variation of this exercise is using a machine designed for it. The machine typically consists of a padded bench for the user to lie on, a roller pad at the bottom for the ankles to rest, and a lever or weight stack to provide resistance.

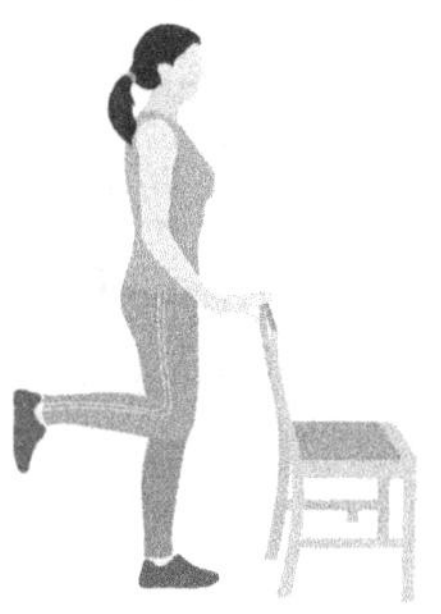

- **Lying leg curl**: Using a weight machine or a resistance band, lie face down on a weight bench with your ankles under a weight or resistance band. Then, curl your legs up toward your glutes and slowly lower them back to the starting position.

- **Seated leg curl:** Using a weight machine, sit on the machine and place your ankles under the roller pad. Then, curl your legs up toward your glutes and slowly lower them back to the starting position.

- **The stability ball hamstring curl:** Lie face down on the ball with your legs extended behind you. Place your hands on the floor for support, then curl your legs up toward your glutes, keeping your knees pointing straight down. Hold for a few counts, then lower your legs to the starting position.

- **The single-leg hamstring curl:** This is a more advanced variation that targets each leg individually. To perform this exercise, lie face down on the machine with one leg extended under the roller pad and the other resting on the bench. Next, curl the extended leg toward your glutes, pause at the peak, and then slowly drop it back to the starting position—repeat for the required reps, then switch legs.

Incorporating the hamstring curl into your workout routine can strengthen your hamstrings, boosting your overall strength training performance and reducing your risk of injury. Keeping your core engaged is essential while performing the curl to maintain stability and prevent excessive lower back arching. As you become stronger, you can gradually increase the number of repetitions to what your muscles can handle.

Knee Extensions

Knee extension exercises are a great way for seniors to improve the strength and stability of their knees. These exercises involve straightening the knee against resistance, which can help to build the knees' supporting muscles and improve overall joint function. But that's not all. Here are some other ways knee extension exercises can help seniors:

- **Improving knee strength:** Knee extension exercises can help strengthen the quadriceps muscles at the front of your thigh. Strong quadriceps muscles can help to support the knee joint, reduce the risk of knee injuries, and improve overall knee function.

- **Improving knee stability:** They can also improve the knee joint's stability, reducing the risk of falls and injuries.

- **Improving knee flexibility:** Knee extension exercises can help improve the knee joint's flexibility, making it easier for seniors to perform daily activities such as standing up, sitting down, and climbing stairs.

- **Reducing pain and discomfort:** Knee extension exercises can help alleviate pain and discomfort in the knee joint, which can benefit seniors with conditions such as osteoarthritis or rheumatoid arthritis.

- **Improving overall physical function:** Strong knee muscles can help support the joints above and below the knee, such as the hips and ankles, improving overall balance and stability. This can help seniors to perform daily activities more quickly and confidently.

To perform knee extensions, follow these steps:

- Sit in a comfortable chair with your feet flat on the floor, shoulder-width apart.

- Slightly raise your hip and bring your right foot forward as you straighten your right knee. Then, hold that position for two to three seconds.

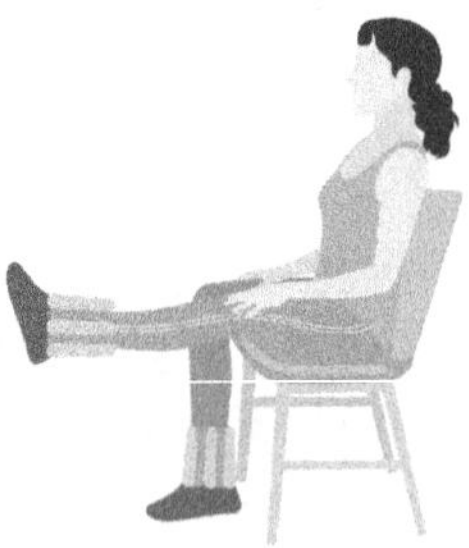

It would help if you did the knee extension exercise for ten repetitions for your right leg, take a short break, then do another ten repetitions for your left leg. That is two sets of ten reps for both legs.

One common variation of knee extension is the leg press machine, and here's how to do it:

- Sit in the machine with your feet on the platform.

- Push the platform away from your body using your legs, straightening your knees as you do so.

- Slowly release the platform back to the starting position and repeat.

The key to making the most from this exercise is to use proper form and start with a lightweight, then gradually increase the weight as your strength improves.

For seniors who may have difficulty with weight-bearing exercises, there are also non-weight-bearing options. And the wall slide is one such exercise. To perform this exercise:

1. Stand with your back to a wall and your feet shoulder-width apart.

2. Slide down the wall slowly until your knees bend at a 90-degree angle.

3. Hold that position for a few seconds, then slowly slide back up the wall to the starting position.

It is important to start with light resistance and a few repetitions and gradually increase as your strength improves. It is also vital to consult with your doctor or physical therapist before beginning any new activity, particularly if you have any pre-existing conditions or injuries.

In addition to knee extension exercises, it's also vital for seniors to maintain overall physical activity and mobility. They can do this by engaging in walking, swimming, or cycling. Stretching and balance exercises are crucial for maintaining flexibility and stability around the knee joint.

In conclusion, knee extension exercises are vital to a senior's overall exercise regimen. These exercises can help to build strength and stability in the knee joint, improving overall mobility and reducing the risk of falls and injuries.

Pelvic Tilts

Pelvic tilts are a simple exercise that can help strengthen the lower back and abdominal area muscles and benefit seniors in many other ways. These benefits include improved strength and flexibility in the lower back and core, improved posture, and reduced pain and discomfort.

As we age, our muscles weaken and become less flexible, leading to pain and discomfort. But as pelvic tilts strengthen and stretch the lower back and core muscles, this can alleviate pain and discomfort. Additionally, pelvic tilts can help improve balance and stability, reducing the risk of falls and injuries.

Another benefit of pelvic tilts for seniors is improved posture. Our posture can become poor as we age due to muscle weakness and gravitational effects. However, pelvic tilts can help to improve posture by strengthening the muscles in the lower back and core, which can help to pull the shoulders back and the chest forward. This can lead to a more upright and confident stance, improving overall appearance and self-esteem.

In addition to the physical benefits, pelvic tilts can improve mental well-being. Many seniors experience pain and discomfort in the lower back and core, which can lead to depression and anxiety. But by performing pelvic tilts, seniors can alleviate pain and discomfort, improving mood and overall well-being.

Pelvic tilts are a low-impact exercise, perfect for older adults with joint pain or arthritis. They also don't require special equipment or gym membership, so they can be done at home.

Ultimately, this exercise helps alleviate back pain, reduce stiffness in the lower back, stretch the back muscles, and strengthen your abdominal and buttock muscles.

To perform pelvic tilts, follow these steps:

- If you can lie on the floor, lie on your back with your legs bent and your feet flat. <u>A firm mattress or even a sofa will suffice.</u>

- Keeping your knees bent and palms faced down next to you, slowly exhale and contract your abdominal muscles, tilting your pelvis upward toward your belly so that your lower back presses into the floor.

- Hold that position for a few seconds, then release and return to the starting position.

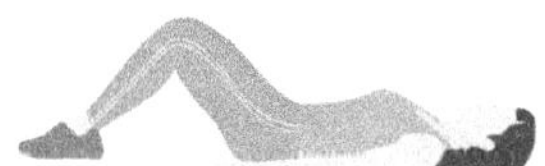

You should do pelvic tilts for ten repetitions and take a short break before doing another ten repetitions. That is, you should do two sets of ten reps.

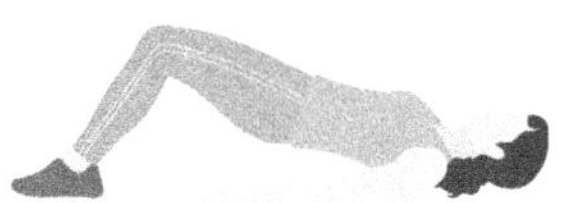

Several variations of the pelvic tilt exercise target slightly different muscles. For example, by tilting your pelvis forward and back, you can work the muscles of your lower back and glutes. Tilting your pelvis to the left and right, you can work the muscles of your obliques (located on the sides of your abdomen).

- **Wall tilts:** You can do pelvic tilts while standing with your back against a wall; if you want to make it more challenging, try adding a resistance band or weight.

Pelvic tilts are excellent for seniors of all fitness levels, as they can be modified to accommodate different abilities. For example, if you're new to exercising, start with a slight tilt and work up to a more significant tilt as you become more comfortable with the movement. But if you're more advanced, you can add weights or resistance bands to the exercise to increase its intensity.

Overall, pelvic tilts are a simple yet effective exercise for anyone looking to strengthen and tone their lower back, hip, and abdominal muscles. They are easy to perform, can be done in various settings, and are suitable for all fitness levels. Incorporating pelvic tilts into your strength training routine can improve your posture, reduce lower back pain, and improve your overall fitness.

Superman/Back Extensions

Back extensions, also known as superman or spinal extensions, involve strengthening the muscles in the back, particularly the lower back. While this exercise is one of the most challenging because it is best performed on the floor, it can benefit seniors in many ways.

One of the primary benefits of back extensions for seniors is improved strength and stability in the lower back. As we age, the muscles in the lower back can become weaker and less flexible, leading to pain and discomfort. Back extensions can help to strengthen and stretch the muscles in the lower back, which can help to alleviate pain and discomfort in this area. Additionally, back extensions can help improve balance and stability, reducing the risk of falls and injuries.

Another benefit of back extensions for seniors is improved posture. Several factors, including muscle weakness, gravity, and inactivity, can cause poor posture. However, back extensions can help improve posture by strengthening the muscles in the lower back, which can help to pull the shoulders back and the chest forward. This can lead to a more upright and confident stance, improving overall appearance and self-esteem.

Back extensions can also help seniors with chronic lower back pain by stretching and strengthening the lower back muscles, reducing stiffness and discomfort. Additionally, back extensions can improve flexibility and range of motion in the lower back, which can help to reduce stiffness and improve mobility.

Back extensions are also beneficial for seniors with osteoporosis. They help strengthen the spine's supporting muscles, which can help to reduce the risk of fractures and injuries. This is an exercise that should be discussed with your physician or your physical therapist. This is a difficult exercise and you should take great care if you do have osteoporosis.

To perform back extensions, follow these steps:

- Lie face down on the floor or a mat with your hands in front of you. You can use one arm at a time or both if you prefer.

- Slowly raise your upper body off the mat like you want to fly, using your lower back muscles to lift your torso.

- Hold the position for about five seconds before lowering your body back to the mat.

Do this movement for ten repetitions, then take a short break before doing another ten repetitions. That is, you should do two sets of ten reps.

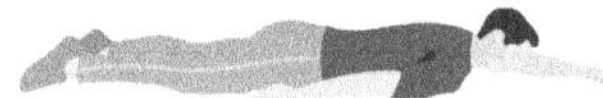

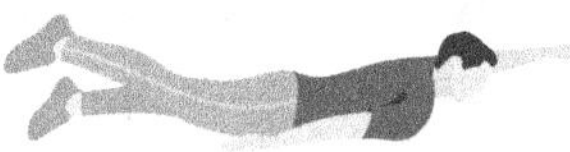

You can also exercise on a firm mattress or couch if you can't lie on the floor. But it's important to keep your lower back in a neutral position and not arch it too much.

The back extension exercise has several variations to target different muscle groups or add variety to your workout routine:

- **Swiss Ball Back Extension:** This variation involves performing the exercise on a stability ball instead of a weight bench. This can increase the difficulty of the movement and target the core muscles more.

- **Supermans:** This exercise targets the lower back and glutes. To perform it, lie face down on a mat with your arms and legs stretched out in front of you. Then, raise your arms and legs simultaneously off the ground, hold for a second, and lower them back down.

- **Weighted Back Extension:** This variation involves holding a weight plate or dumbbell against your chest while performing the exercise. This can increase the intensity and help build more strength in your lower back.

- **Hyperextensions:** This exercise targets the lower back, glutes, and hamstrings. Start by positioning yourself face down on a hyperextension bench, with your hips just off the edge. Then, slowly lower your torso toward the ground and lift it back up to the starting position.

- **Good Mornings:** This exercise targets the lower back, glutes, and hamstrings. To perform it, stand with your feet shoulder-width apart and your knees slightly bent. Then, holding a barbell behind your neck, bend forward at the hips while keeping your back straight and returning to your starting point.

Note that it's essential to use proper form when performing back extension exercises, and recommended to consult the machine's instructions or ask a trainer for guidance if you are at the gym. Adding lower body exercises to your routine is important, so aim to perform these strength training exercises at least two days per week. Also, I need to emphasize the importance of starting with a lower intensity and gradually increasing it as you progress.

In conclusion, exercising the lower body is vital for overall fitness and well-being. Working the large muscle groups of the legs and hips can improve cardiovascular health, increase strength, and flexibility, and promote and maintain a youthful appearance.

Key Takeaways

- Exercising the lower body can positively affect mental well-being. Regular exercise improves mood, reduces stress and anxiety, and promotes overall mental health.

- Hamstring curls can help to improve your running, jumping, and reflexes, making them essential exercises for athletes and sports enthusiasts.

- Knee extension exercises can help strengthen the quadriceps muscles at the front of your thigh.

- Back extensions can help to strengthen and stretch the muscles in the lower back, which can help to alleviate pain and discomfort in this area.

- Strong knee muscles can help support the joints above and below the knee, such as the hips and ankles, improving overall balance and stability.

- Hamstring curls also engage and strengthen the core muscles and glutes.

- Pelvic tilts help to strengthen and stretch the muscles in the lower back and core, which can help to alleviate pain and discomfort in these areas.

- Back extensions can help to improve posture by strengthening the muscles in the lower back, which can help to pull the shoulders back and the chest forward.

CHAPTER 7: COOLING DOWN!

"The miracle isn't that I finished. The miracle is that I had the courage to start."

– John Bingham

Cooling down is as important as warming up because exercising helps your body recover safely and effectively. Simply put, a cool-down involves those physical activities you should perform at the end of your strength training workout or exercise session.

The goal of a cool-down is to gradually return your heart rate, body temperature, and blood pressure levels to normal before continuing your routine. Cooling down after a workout has many benefits, some of which are listed below:

- **Improving flexibility and range of motion: Cool-down exercises can improve flexibility and range of motion by helping the muscles to relax and release tension. You can experience these benefits when you perform stretches targeting major muscle groups. The best time to work on your flexibility is when your body is warm, and you're breaking a sweat.**

Instead of jumping off the treadmill and straight into a toe touch, experts recommend completing some dynamic stretches first. This can lower your chance of injury, alleviate back pain, and boost sports performance. Spending enough time on this cool-down exercise will also improve your flexibility and mobility, which may help you avoid muscle tears, back pain, and joint problems.

- **Reducing the risk of injury:** Cool-down exercises can help to reduce the risk of injury by gradually decreasing the heart rate, blood pressure, and body temperature. Sprains, strains, and tears in the lower back, hip flexors, knees, hamstrings, and quadriceps are some of the most common injuries these exercises can help you avoid.

So, focus on elongating your muscle fibers, which were under tension during your workout, to achieve your entire range of motion. Activities that focus on the cardiovascular system include walking, jogging, or stretching, and you can always do anyone after a strength training workout.

- **Improving recovery:** Cool-down exercises can also improve recovery by reducing muscle soreness and stiffness and restoring the body's natural balance. You can achieve this by performing exercises focusing on the muscles used during your workout or your cardiovascular system.

- **Improving overall health and fitness:** Cool-down exercises can also help to improve overall health and wellness by allowing the body to recover and restore itself after a workout. As in the previous point, you can achieve this with exercises targeting your cardiovascular system or the muscles you use while exercising.

Now that you understand the importance of cooling down let's explore the different cool-down exercises you can do.

Upper Stretches

Upper body stretches are essential to maintaining flexibility and mobility for seniors. Our muscles and joints can become stiffer as we age, making it harder to perform everyday activities. However, upper body stretches offer several benefits for seniors:

- **Increased flexibility:** Stretching your upper body muscles can help to increase flexibility and range of motion in your arms, back, and shoulders, which can make it easier to perform daily activities such as reaching and lifting a load.

- **Improved posture:** Upper body tightness can contribute to poor posture, leading to back and neck pain. However, stretching can assist in relaxing tense muscles and improving alignment, resulting in better posture.

- **Reduced pain and stiffness:** Stretching can help reduce pain and stiffness in the upper body by releasing muscle tension. This can be especially beneficial for seniors experiencing chronic pain or stiffness due to arthritis.

- **Increased circulation:** Stretching can help increase blood flow to the muscles, speeding up recovery from an injury or surgery and promoting overall health.

- **Better balance and coordination:** Stretching the upper body can also help improve balance and coordination, reducing the risk of falls.

Here are upper body stretches you can do:

- **Shoulder roll:** Stand with your arms at your sides and rotate your shoulders forward, up, back, and down in a circular motion. Repeat for several rotations.

- **Chest stretch:**

  - Stand in a doorway with your arms at shoulder level, gripping the doorframe.

  - Step forward and push your chest out.

○ Hold for 15-30 seconds.

- **Tricep stretch:** Raise your right arm above your head and bend your elbow, so your hand is behind your head. Then, use your left hand to gently press down on your right elbow, feeling the stretch in your right tricep.

- **Bicep stretch:** Stand with your arms at your sides. Reach up and clasp your hands together with your palms facing down. As I mentioned earlier, upper body tightness can contribute to poor posture, leading to back and neck pain. However, stretching can help relax tense muscles and improve alignment, resulting in better posture.

Stretching before and after any physical activity is vital to prevent injury and improve flexibility. It's also important to breathe deeply and never force a stretch.

In addition, seniors need to perform upper body stretches under the supervision of a healthcare professional, especially if they have any pre-existing medical conditions. This can help prevent injury and ensure that the stretches are tailored to their needs.

Calf/Hamstring Stretch

For seniors and the elderly, hamstring stretching is crucial to lower back and leg flexibility. As we age, our lower body stiffens, and our arms and shoulders lose their former wide range of motion.

As a result, putting on our shoes and socks will become more difficult. This reduced range of motion will also affect our functional mobility, such as standing up from a chair, side-stepping around a table, or reaching over to pick up dropped mail. This is what makes hamstring stretching so important. But what benefits do hamstring stretching offer seniors, exactly?

- **Improved flexibility:** Hamstrings are a group of muscles in the back of the thigh that can become tight with age. But stretching them can help improve flexibility and range of motion in the legs.

- **Reduced risk of injury:** Tight hamstrings can increase seniors' risk of falls and other injuries, which stretching can help them avoid.

- **Pain relief:** Tight hamstrings can also cause lower back and knee pain, which can reduce when you stretch these muscles.

- **Improved posture:** Tight hamstrings can cause the pelvis to tilt forward, leading to poor posture. Fortunately, stretching them can help correct this defect and improve overall posture.

- **Improved balance:** Tight hamstrings can make it more challenging to maintain balance. However, stretching them can improve balance and stability.

- **Improved physical function:** Tight hamstrings can make it harder to perform daily activities like walking and climbing stairs. However, stretching your hamstrings can improve physical function and make it easier to perform these tasks.

To do upper stretches, follow these steps:

- Stand facing a sturdy chair.

- Lean over your chair with your elbows slightly bent; you should feel a pull in your legs.

- If you don't, bend your elbows more.

- Hold that position for about twenty seconds, then relax and repeat the exercise as many times as necessary.

Below are some variations of the hamstring stretch:

- **Standing hamstring stretch:** For this variation, stand with your feet hip-width apart and bend forward from the hips, reaching your hands toward your toes. Keep your knees slightly bent to focus on stretching the hamstrings.

- **Seated hamstring stretch:** To perform this exercise, sit on the floor with one leg extended in front of you and the other leg bent with the foot against the inner thigh of the extended leg. Then, lean forward from the hips to stretch the hamstring of the extended leg.

- **Lunges hamstring stretch:** To perform this exercise, step forward with one leg and bend both knees to lower your body. Then, keep the back leg straight and your back heel lifted to stretch the hamstring of the back leg.

- **Butterfly stretch:** Sit on the floor with the soles of your feet together, and your knees bent. Then, gently press your knees toward the floor to stretch your inner thigh and hamstrings.

- **Straddle stretch:** For this variation, sit on the floor with your legs wide apart and reach forward to touch your toes. Then, keep your back straight to stretch the inner thigh and hamstrings.

- **Reclining hand-to-toe stretch:** To perform this variation, lie on your back, extend one leg straight up and reach toward the toes of that leg with your hands. Keep the other leg flat on the floor and hold the stretch for the desired time.

It is important to stretch correctly and use proper form to avoid injury. It is also recommended to consult a personal trainer or physical therapist before starting a stretching regimen, particularly for seniors or people with underlying health conditions.

Quad Stretch

The quadriceps (also known as the quads) are a group of four muscles located at the front of the thigh. They are responsible for straightening the knee we use in walking, climbing stairs, and standing up from a seated position.

We rely on our quadriceps to perform many daily duties, and if we spend a lot of time sitting, they might get tight.

While extending the quadriceps seems easy to prevent them from getting tight, the quadriceps can be difficult to stretch. This is because you have to bring your knee up and balance on one leg, which might be difficult if you have mobility limitations in your knee or shoulder or have balance concerns.

Regardless of your fitness level, the quadriceps are an important area of the body to stretch and should be a primary focus. Quad stretches are essential for seniors to maintain mobility, flexibility, and balance.

As we age, our quadriceps muscles can tighten and weaken, leading to an increased risk of falls, knee pain, and difficulty with daily activities. But by performing quad stretches regularly, seniors can maintain the strength and flexibility of these muscles, improving overall mobility and quality of life.

One of the main benefits of quad stretches for seniors is improved balance. The quadriceps muscles play a major role in maintaining a stable upright position and providing support for the knee. So when they are tight and weak, it can lead to an unstable gait and an increased risk of falls. By stretching the quads, seniors can improve the strength and flexibility of these muscles, improving their balance and reducing the risk of falls.

Another benefit of quad stretches for seniors is reduced knee pain. The quadriceps muscles are closely connected to the knee joint, and tightness in these muscles can lead to pain and inflammation in the knee. But by stretching the quads, seniors can alleviate tension in the knee joint and reduce pain and discomfort. Additionally, stretching the quads can help improve the knee's range of motion, hugely benefiting seniors with arthritis or other conditions that can limit mobility.

Quad stretches can also help to improve posture and alignment. Our bodies become less flexible as we age, and we may develop poor posture. And when the quadriceps muscles are tight, they can pull the pelvis forward, causing the spine to curve and the shoulders to round forward.

However, by stretching the quads, seniors can help realign their pelvis and spine, improving posture and reducing the risk of back pain.

Quad stretches can also help to relieve pain and discomfort associated with arthritis. Arthritis is a common condition among seniors, which can cause pain and stiffness in the joints. However, stretching the quadriceps muscles can help to alleviate tension in the knee joint and reduce pain associated with arthritis. Additionally, stretching the quads can help improve the knee's range of motion, making it easier for seniors with arthritis to move around and perform daily activities.

Follow these simple and effective procedures to stretch your quadriceps easily:

- Place yourself behind a firm chair.

- Bend one knee and reach it with your hand. If you can't reach it, pull up as much as possible.

- Hold that position for about twenty seconds, then relax and repeat the exercise as many times as necessary.

- Do the same for the opposite knee.

Below are some variations of the quad stretch you can do:

1, Dynamic Stretch

Dynamic stretches are movement-based stretching in which the muscles are employed to achieve a stretch. Here's how to go about it:

- Stand tall, with your shoulders pulled back and down and your feet hip-width apart.

- Bring your foot up behind you as far as you feel comfortable, then lower it.

- Repeat this with the other leg.

- Continue to alternate legs for the duration of the exercise.

2. Side-lying stretch

Here's how to do this exercise:

- Lie on your side on your bed, sofa, or floor in the most comfortable posture for you.

- Bring your ankle to your buttocks while pulling your foot with your arm.

- Pull the resistance band or belt gently until you feel a stretch in your quadriceps.

- Make sure your leg is straight up and not pointing in or out.

- Hold that position for a specified time before repeating the exercise on the opposite leg.

Finally, quad stretches can improve your overall performance if you engage in sports like golf, swimming, etc. When the quadriceps muscles are tight, they can limit the range of motion and reduce power output. But by stretching the quads, seniors can improve the flexibility and strength of these muscles, boosting their athletic performance and reducing the risk of injury.

In conclusion, the quadriceps muscles play a key role in maintaining a stable upright position and supporting the knee. So seniors can use quad stretches to improve the strength and flexibility of their quadriceps, improving their balance, posture, and athletic performance and reducing the risk of falls, knee pain, and the pain and discomfort associated with arthritis. Seniors need to consult their healthcare provider before beginning a new exercise routine, but quad stretches should be a regular exercise routine once cleared.

Neck and Shoulder Stretch

Stretching is important for maintaining physical health and mobility, especially for seniors. One of the primary benefits of neck and shoulder stretches for seniors is that they can help to improve the range of motion. Our muscles and joints can become stiff and inflexible as we age, making it difficult to move freely and comfortably. Regular stretching can help to loosen up these tight areas, allowing seniors to move more efficiently and with less pain. Stretching can also help reduce inflammation and pain in damaged joints, which is especially good for seniors with arthritis.

Another benefit of neck and shoulder stretches for seniors is that they can help to reduce pain and stiffness. Many seniors experience pain and discomfort in their neck and shoulders, often due to poor posture or prolonged sitting or standing. However, stretching can loosen tight muscles and release tension, reducing pain and stiffness. This can be especially beneficial for seniors who suffer from severe conditions, such as fibromyalgia or chronic fatigue syndrome.

In addition to improving the range of motion and reducing pain and stiffness, neck and shoulder stretches can also help to increase flexibility. Flexibility is an essential aspect of overall physical health, especially for seniors. Our muscles and joints become less flexible as we age, making us more susceptible to injury. Regular stretching can help to slow down this process and maintain flexibility, even as we age. This can be especially beneficial for seniors recovering from an injury or surgery, as it can help prevent further damage and promote healing.

Neck and shoulder stretch can also help improve balance and coordination, which are important for maintaining independence and preventing falls. In addition, stretching can improve the range of motion and flexibility in the neck and shoulders, which improves overall balance and coordination.

Simple neck and shoulder stretches you can do are:

- Clasp your hands and push out forward. Hold about twenty seconds, relax, and repeat as necessary.

- **The seated neck roll:** Sit comfortably in a chair with your feet on the floor to perform this stretch. Then, slowly drop your right ear to your right shoulder, feeling the stretch in the left side of the neck. Hold that position for ten seconds before repeating it on the opposite side of your body.

- **The shoulder roll:** Stand with your feet hip-width apart and your arms by your sides to do this stretch. Slowly roll your shoulders forward, up, and back, feeling the stretch in your shoulders and upper back. Hold this position for ten seconds, then repeat it in the opposite direction.

- **The arm across the chest stretch:** Raise your right arm across your chest and hold it with your left hand. Gently pull your right arm toward your chest and hold for a count of ten. Repeat on other side.

- **Seated spinal twist:** Sit comfortably in a chair with your feet flat on the floor. Hold your right hand on the back of the chair and gently twist your torso to the right, feeling the stretch in your spine and shoulders. Hold for a count of ten, then repeat on the other side.

Remember that stretching should be done slowly and gently, without bouncing or forcing the body into uncomfortable positions. It's also important to breathe deeply and relax your stretching muscles. Stretching should never cause pain; if it does, stop immediately.

Consult a doctor or physical therapist before starting any new exercise program, particularly if you have any pre-existing medical conditions or injuries. They can help you develop a stretching program tailored to your needs and abilities.

Stretching exercises for the neck and shoulders are necessary to maintain flexibility and range of motion as we age. So, incorporating these stretches into your daily routine can help alleviate stiffness and pain, improve mobility, and enhance your overall quality of life. Always warm up before stretching, stretch slowly and gently, breathe deeply, and relax the stretched muscles.

In summary, cool-down exercises are valuable for anyone performing strength training activities. They help to decrease the heart rate and breathing rate. They also facilitate blood flow to the muscles, which helps prevent blood from gathering around one spot in your legs. That way, the chances of getting injured and the stress on your heart and other muscles will reduce.

Cooling down also helps to reduce muscle soreness and stiffness, improve flexibility and range of motion, and improve recovery and overall health and fitness. To maximize benefits, you should include 5-10 minutes of cool-down exercises after a workout or physical activity.

Key Takeaways

- Cool-down gradually helps to return your heart rate, body temperature, and blood pressure levels to normal before continuing your everyday routine.

- Cool-down exercises can also help to improve overall health and fitness by allowing the body to recover and restore itself after a workout.

- Stretching the upper body can help improve balance and coordination, reducing the risk of falls.

- Regardless of your fitness level, the quadriceps are a crucial area of the body to stretch and should be noticed. Quad stretches are an important exercise for seniors to maintain mobility, flexibility, and balance.

- Neck and shoulder stretches can help improve balance and coordination, which is essential for maintaining independence and preventing falls.

- Cool-down exercises can help to reduce muscle soreness and stiffness by gradually allowing the muscles to return to their pre-exercise state. You can perform stretches and exercises focusing on the muscles during the workout.

- Tight hamstrings can increase seniors' risk of falls and other injuries. However, stretching them can help prevent these types of injuries.

- Spending enough time doing cool-down exercises will improve your flexibility and mobility, which may help you avoid muscle tears, back pain, and joint problems.

- Upper body tightness can contribute to poor posture and back and neck pain. Stretching can assist in relaxing tense muscles and improving alignment, resulting in better posture.

- Neck and shoulder stretching can help to loosen up these tight areas, allowing seniors to move more efficiently and with less pain.

- Quad stretches can also help to relieve pain and discomfort associated with arthritis, a common condition among seniors, which can cause pain and stiffness in the joints.

- By stretching the quads, seniors can improve the flexibility and strength of these muscles, improving their athletic performance and reducing the risk of injury.

Chapter 8: Final Nuggets of Information

"It's easier to stay in shape if you never let yourself get out of shape in the first place."

– Bill Loguidice

It could occur after a period of indulgence—the winter holidays or a summer vacation trip—or gradually, after spending too much time on the sofa and at the refrigerator. But when you look in the mirror, you scarcely recognize yourself now. Maybe you're getting older.

Have you put on any weight or experienced muscle tone loss? Is your posture sagging, or do you look tired or even depressed? These are telltale symptoms that it's time to pay attention to your physical health. But what if you need to prepare for this forthcoming fitness revolution properly?

Of course, before commencing any workout regimen, you should always consult with your doctor. Then, once you do that, the next thing to do is to choose your fitness venue; whether you prefer your home or a gym, you want a venue that caters to all your fitness needs. If you decide to use a gym, choose one with educated and helpful trainers with varying personalities so you can choose the one that best matches your own. All equipment must be up to date, and the level of cleanliness must be good.

It would help if you also concentrate on your diet and nutrition. Also, learn the importance of various macronutrients such as carbohydrates, proteins, and, yes, even fats. Begin to grasp the hydration process and how to provide your body with enough water to function effectively. You'll also need to dress appropriately during your workouts. For instance, you could wear wicking tops, bottoms, and athletic shoes with adequate support; you could also carry a gym bag with amenities, towels, drink, and snacks. Finally, you must stick to your program, strive for your fitness objectives, and keep a positive mindset.

No Matter Your Fitness Level, It's Never Too Late to Start

No matter your current fitness level, there is always time to start working toward a healthier, more active lifestyle. Whether you are a beginner or a seasoned athlete looking to make a comeback, there are steps you can take to begin your fitness journey.

First, set realistic goals. For instance, expecting to run a marathon in a few months may be unrealistic if you are a beginner. Instead, start by setting small, achievable goals such as going for a walk every day or completing a set number of push-ups. Then, as you progress, you can gradually increase the intensity and duration of your workouts.

Second, find an activity that you enjoy. You are less likely to commit to an activity you don't like. So, try different activities such as swimming, cycling, dancing, or weightlifting to find something you enjoy. Additionally, you can work out with a friend or a personal trainer to make it more fun and motivating.

Third, be patient with yourself. Remember that you didn't get to your current fitness level overnight, and you won't get to your desired fitness level overnight, either. It takes time and effort to see results, so don't compare yourself to others. Everyone's journey is different, so focus on your progress.

The fourth step is to seek professional help if needed. If you have any health concerns or injuries, it is always a good idea to consult a doctor or physical therapist before starting a new exercise routine. They can help you create a safe and effective workout plan that considers your individual needs.

Knowing where to start can be difficult for people who have been away from fitness training for a long time. But remember that there is always time to start working toward a healthier, more active lifestyle. You can start by setting small, achievable goals, finding an activity you enjoy, being consistent, being patient with yourself, and seeking professional help.

For those who were working on becoming fit, then stopped, remember that it is not a failure. It is normal to take a break or experience a setback. But the most important thing is to pick yourself up and start again with renewed motivation and a new mindset.

Remember that everyone's journey is different, so the most important thing is to take the first step and keep moving forward.

Exercising Increases Your Mood, Mind, and Memory

One of the most notable benefits of exercising is its positive impact on mood, mind, and memory. Regular exercise has been shown to reduce symptoms of depression and anxiety, improve cognitive function and memory, and even slow down the progression of certain diseases such as Alzheimer's.

Exercise improves mood by releasing endorphins, also known as "feel-good" hormones. Endorphins interact with the brain's receptors that control pain and emotions, leading to an overall sense of well-being and happiness. Additionally, exercise can reduce stress levels by decreasing the amount of the stress hormone cortisol in the body.

Exercise also plays a critical role in cognitive function and memory. Research has shown that regular physical activity can improve attention, focus, and problem-solving skills. It also has a positive impact on the hippocampus, the part of the brain that is responsible for memory and spatial navigation. Studies have also found that people who exercise regularly tend to have a better overall cognitive function and a lower risk of developing conditions such as dementia and Alzheimer's.

In addition to these benefits, regular exercise improves sleep quality, boosting mood, mind, and memory. When we sleep well, our brain can consolidate, and process information gathered that day, which helps to improve memory and cognitive function.

Pay Attention to Your Health

Seniors need to pay attention to their health when exercising because as we age, our body's ability to recover from injury or strain decreases. Additionally, older adults may have underlying health conditions that need attention when starting an exercise routine.

Here are a few tips for seniors to pay attention to their health when exercising:

- **Please consult with a healthcare professional:** Before starting any exercise program, seniors need to consult with their healthcare provider to ensure it's safe. The healthcare provider can then recommend the best exercises for their specific health conditions.

- **Start slowly:** It is important for seniors to start with a low-intensity exercise program and gradually increase the intensity and duration over time. This will help prevent injury and make the transition to regular exercise much easier.

- **Focus on balance and flexibility:** As we age, the risk of falls increases, so it is essential for seniors to include exercises that improve balance and flexibility in their routines. These can include yoga, Tai chi, and balance exercises using a stability ball.

- **Listen to your body:** Seniors need to pay attention to how they feel during and after exercise. If they experience pain or discomfort, they should stop the exercise and consult their healthcare provider. If you are sick or injured or your muscles feel unusually sore, STOP immediately. It is OK to take care of yourself.

- **Always do what you can:** If the plan tells you to do twenty reps, and you can only do ten, that is OK! The recommended repetitions are simply that—recommendations, not hard and fast rules. So you can constantly adjust them to your taste. You can also add additional weights if you feel the ones you use are too light.

- **Stay hydrated:** Seniors need to drink plenty of water before, during, and after exercising to stay hydrated and prevent dehydration.

- **Get enough rest:** As we age, our bodies require more rest and recovery time. So, seniors need to make sure they are getting enough sleep and allowing their bodies to recover after exercise.

In essence, you need to pay attention to your health when exercising by consulting with a healthcare professional, starting slowly, focusing on balance and flexibility, incorporating strength training, listening to your body, staying hydrated, and getting enough rest. This will ensure that your exercise routine is safe and effective to help you achieve your fitness goals.

You're on the Path to Rewriting Your Fitness Journey

Rewriting your fitness journey can be a challenging and rewarding process. It involves taking a step back to evaluate your current approach to fitness and making changes to achieve your desired results. Once you set your goals, the next step is to create a plan to achieve them. This plan should include both exercise and nutrition components. When it comes to exercise, it is important to choose activities that you enjoy that also align with your goals. For example, if your goal is to lose weight, include cardio and strength training in your exercise plan. If your goal is to improve your overall health and well-being, consider including activities such as yoga or meditation.

When it comes to nutrition, focus on whole, nutrient-dense foods. You can eat fruits, vegetables, lean proteins, and whole grains, pay attention to portion sizes and avoid processed foods and added sugars. A registered dietitian can help you create a personalized nutrition plan that aligns with your goals and lifestyle.

It is also essential to make sure you are consistent in your efforts. Consistency is the key to making progress and achieving your goals. And stick to your exercise and nutrition plan, even when it gets tough, or you feel unmotivated. To stay on track, try to make fitness and healthy eating habits a part of your daily routine.

Another aspect of rewriting your fitness journey is tracking your progress. You can see how far you have come and identify areas where you need adjustments. You can track your progress by measuring your weight, body measurements, and strength or endurance. You can also take progress photos and journal your workouts and meals.

As you track your progress, you may need to adjust your plan to achieve your goals. For instance, if you are losing weight slower than you would like, you may need to raise the intensity or duration of your workouts or make dietary changes. To reach your goals, you must be adaptable and alter your approach as needed.

You must follow your doctor's recovery instructions if you are diagnosed with significant sports or fitness-related injuries. Muscles, tendons, and ligaments can take longer to heal than bones. So, ensure you don't skip or minimize any physical therapy sessions; if your doctor recommends home exercises, do them for the entire duration.

It would help if you also tried to figure out what caused the injury and do your best to prevent it from happening again. If you forgot to warm up, overtrained, or attempted a tricky maneuver without a trainer's guidance, you can avoid these scenarios in the future. If you took a wrong step, had a cramp, or fell, those are not things you could have changed. Accepting this and moving on is critical. Once your doctor or physical therapist clears you to return to the gym, make sure you follow these tips for an easy reentry:

- **Make a strategy:** Create an exercise-based rehab plan with your doctor, physiotherapist, or trainer. Your physical therapist or trainer will also be able to detect any improper movements or muscle imbalances that could cause future problems.

- **Stay fueled:** You must eat well and stay hydrated during rehabilitation and reentry. So, avoid alcohol, refined sugar, and white flour; instead, focus on lean protein, complex carbohydrates, and plenty of greens.

- **Allow yourself plenty of time:** Even if you start to feel like your pre-injury self again, stick to your recovery regimen for at least another two weeks as you continue to gain strength. Once your rehab requirements have been adjusted, you can focus on workouts that stress stability, flexibility, and core strength.

- **Roll with it:** It's vital to warm up your injured muscles before exercising, so use a foam roller to massage the sore areas of your body.

Now that you are training regularly, you can rewrite your fitness journey. Your balance will improve, your energy will increase, and you will mostly build confidence as you gain mobility. It is essential to stick with your plan, but as we know, life can often get in the way!

Vacation, work, and illness can put a speed bump in our path. But even if this happens, don't quit! All you have to do is restart. Remember why you got this book in the first place.

Key Takeaways

- Whether you choose your home or a gym, you want a fitness venue that caters to all your fitness needs.

- No matter your current fitness level, there is always time to start working toward a healthier, more active lifestyle.

- Regular exercise can reduce symptoms of depression and anxiety, improve cognitive function and memory, and even slow the progression of certain diseases such as Alzheimer's.

- Seniors need to start with a low-intensity exercise program and gradually increase the intensity and duration over time. This will help them prevent injury and make the transition to regular exercise much more effortless.

- As we age, our bodies require more rest and recovery time. Seniors need to make sure they are getting enough sleep and allowing their bodies to recover after exercise.

- The first step to rewriting your fitness journey is to set clear and specific goals. Define what you want to achieve in your health, fitness, and well-being. Your goals should be measurable, so you can track your progress and adjust your plan as needed.

Chapter 9: Create Your Personal Fitness Journey

"You dream. You plan. You reach. There will be obstacles. There will be doubters. There will be mistakes. But with hard work, with belief, with confidence and trust in yourself and those around you, there are no limits."

– Michael Phelps

The fundamentals and principles of strength training activity design are the same regardless of the trainee's age. But because the functional capacity of many seniors varies, the best program for each is individualized to meet their needs and medical concerns.

Currently, periodized training works best in several situations when training older adults. As with any untrained population, advanced program design is not required to produce positive results in the early training phases. When a senior's long-term strength training goal progresses toward higher levels of muscular strength, research supports the use of variation in the strength training program.

However, always introduce progression at a gradual pace to avoid acute injury and allow time for adaptation. As I explained in the previous chapter, creating your fitness journey requires you to consider your health and pay attention to specific medical aspects, such as cardiovascular problems and arthritis. Some seniors may need an introductory conditioning period before training with more intense programs.

Performance Evaluation

To determine training progress and personalize the program for yourself, evaluate your strength (on the equipment used in training, if you're using one), muscle endurance, functional ability (e.g., your ability to lift a chair, get off a chair, etc.), nutrition, and quality of life.

The American College of Sports Medicine (ACSM) recommends that when implementing a strength training program, you should consult a physician before strength training to determine if they need any other testing for any medical condition.

Muscle strength is one of the most common factors for measuring strength training performance and can be measured using a dynamometer or hand-held muscle tester to assess the amount of force a muscle can produce. For example, a dynamometer can measure the strength of the quadriceps muscle by having the senior perform a knee extension exercise.

Another important factor for measuring strength training performance is muscle endurance. This is measured by counting the number of repetitions of a specific exercise a person can perform or by measuring the time it takes them to complete a set number of repetitions. For example, a senior might perform a set of ten bicep curls and the number of repetitions they can perform before reaching fatigue.

Physical function is another important aspect of strength training performance for seniors. This is evaluated using tests such as the Timed Up and Go test, which measures the time it takes a person to rise from a chair, walk a short distance, and return to the chair. This test can provide insight into a senior's ability to perform activities of daily living and can be used to track progress over time.

Quality of life is also an essential aspect of performance evaluation for strength training for seniors. Surveys and questionnaires can assess how strength training impacts a senior's overall quality of life, including their ability to perform daily activities. For example, a senior might be asked to rate their ability to perform climbing stairs or carry groceries before and after participating in a strength training program.

It is also important to note that seniors may have different strength training goals than other age groups. For example, many seniors may not be as concerned with building muscle mass as they are with maintaining or improving their physical function. This is why it's essential for strength training programs for seniors to be tailored to their specific goals and needs.

Another consideration when evaluating the performance of a strength training program for seniors is safety. Many seniors may have underlying health conditions or are at risk of specific injuries. So, strength training programs need to be designed and implemented to minimize the risk of injury and consider any limitations or restrictions that a senior may have.

One important cautionary note concerning strength testing is that adequate familiarization with strength testing is necessary for gaining accurate information. Strength assessment does have a potential age-related need for more significant numbers of familiarization sessions with maximal strength testing. Without adequate familiarization, some of the dramatically high percentage gains in strength for seniors may be due to learning effects on how to perform the exercise with heavier loads.

Proper exercise technique is vital to safely implementing a strength training program. Many have the misconception that machines are safer than free weights. With machines, people often push longer and strain harder with repetition, even when the technique fails, causing strains or muscle pulls. People can avoid injuries by using free-weight exercises because of the need for balance and control in multiple planes of motion, which prevents the continuation of a movement if the proper technique is misused. Thus, when seniors implement a program, technique training and supervision in a strength training program for machines and free weights are sometimes lost

Needs Analysis

People respond differently to a given strength training program based on their current training status, past training experience, and response to the training stress. When you develop a strength training program, consider pretesting, setting individualized goals, designing a program, and developing evaluation methods. Competent supervision is also essential for optimizing strength and conditioning programs (e.g., the National Strength and Conditioning Association's [NSCA]) in the United States.

There is now also a Special Population NSCA certification that includes training the elderly to identify minimal competence, which is considered prudent for those working with this population. In older adults, strength training should be part of a lifelong fitness lifestyle, so continual reevaluations of program goals and designs are necessary for optimal results and adherence.

The American College of Sports Medicine has advised that people who start an exercise program be classified into one of three risk categories:

- Healthy, less than one coronary risk factor (hypertension or smoking) or cardiopulmonary or metabolic disease.

- At higher risk, more than two coronary risk factors or cardiopulmonary or metabolic disease symptoms.

- Previously diagnosed with conditions such as cardiovascular, pulmonary, or metabolic disease.

As noted by the American College of Sports Medicine concerning coronary vascular disease (CVD) and coronary heart disease (CHD), as well as other risks, consultation with a medical specialist and diagnostic exercise testing should be undertaken when medically required and, by clinical practice guidelines, based on indications and symptoms of the disease.

Exercise under an experienced fitness expert's guidance can improve adherence and reduce the risk of exercise in persons at high risk of unfavorable CHD events. Seniors, particularly rookie exercisers and those with health concerns or disabilities, will most likely benefit from consulting a well-trained fitness professional.

Routine Frequency

A significant concern for seniors regarding strength training is proper progression to avoid injury or acute overuse. We might speculate that seniors' muscles require more extended recovery periods between exercise sessions. Therefore, you want to vary the intensity and volume of your workout to ensure recovery, especially after workouts where significant muscle damage has occurred because of heavy resistances or high volumes.

Care is needed not to "overshoot" the physiological ability to repair tissues after a workout. As in all age groups, proper nutritional intake and rest are necessary for recovery.

The frequency at which you perform each type of program is important, as it can impact the effectiveness of the training and your overall health and fitness. When designing a strength training program for seniors, it is crucial to consider the appropriate workout frequency to ensure optimal results.

The American College of Sports Medicine (ACSM) recommends that seniors engage in strength training at least twice per week, with a minimum of forty-eight hours between each workout to allow muscle recovery. This break allows for adequate muscle recovery and repair time, essential for muscle growth and strength gain.

In my recovery, I started my strength training only two days a week and built up to four days a week. This gave me a broader range of options for designing a program that worked for me. If the number of sets is balanced, two weekly training sessions may be as efficient as four for seniors. It is your choice to make.

However, it's also important to note that the workout frequency can vary depending on the individual's fitness level, health conditions, and goals. For example, seniors new to strength training or who have been sedentary for an extended period may benefit from starting with one workout per week and gradually increasing the frequency as they become more comfortable and confident with the exercises.

Additionally, seniors with certain health conditions, such as osteoarthritis, may benefit from a lower workout frequency or focus on exercises that target specific muscle groups. In these cases, it's essential to consult a healthcare professional or a certified fitness professional to ensure that the workout frequency and exercises are appropriate for the individual's health conditions.

Choice of Exercise

With any equipment, taking care of yourself helps you attain a good range of motion and safely controls the resistance throughout the full range of motion. Seniors may need to supplement strength exercise training with mobility training to achieve their full range of motion. In the absence of physical limitations, however, the chosen exercise may not differ from that of any other person except for decreased volume.

It is important to focus primarily on all major muscle groups over a week. You want to mix and match routines to build your plan.

Pop squats, pelvic tilts, and similar multi-joint or compound movements can help to increase bone mineral density in sedentary, post-menopausal women between ages forty-five and sixty-five. Therefore, including these exercises in programs for older women seems warranted.

As described earlier, upper body exercise and exercises that stimulate muscles attached at primary bone sites of concern may increase spinal bone density. As the program progresses, the progression of exercises should activate as much of the skeletal muscle mass as possible to facilitate adaptation. In addition, heavy weights may not be appropriate for twisting and turning movements. Exercises incorporating these movements help develop functional abilities better than linear ones.

The exercise equipment must fit your individual and functional capacity; some machines are too large, have too much initial resistance, or have inappropriate load increments for some seniors. Free weights, isokinetic machines, pneumatic machines, and stack plate machines have all been used. Isokinetic, pneumatics, or hydraulics allow easier initiations of the exercise movement and a smoother strength progression than standard machines.

Order of Exercise

When it comes to the order of your exercise routine, you want to start with warm-ups and then large-muscle-group exercises at the beginning of the workout. This placement will reduce fatigue and help you use higher intensities or greater resistances in these exercises.

Optimal stimulation of large muscle groups in the lower extremities (e.g., with the back extensions) and the upper body (e.g., with the wall push-ups) should be a top priority in programs for seniors. Small muscle group exercises and cool-down activities follow large muscle group exercises when you do total body workouts, rotating exercises between the upper and lower body and between opposing muscle groups.

In addition, the rest between sets and exercises dictates the metabolic intensity of a resistance training workout. In seniors, tolerance of anaerobic acidic conditions is less than in younger people. Typically, you can take rest periods of two to three minutes between sets and exercises. But you should carefully check for any symptoms (e.g., nausea, dizziness) and change the program once you notice any.

Tolerance of the workout is paramount for optimal training. Rest periods that are too short can also produce a drastic reduction in the load used in successive sets if recovery is not sufficient before the next set or exercise is initiated. Short rest intervals enhance local muscular endurance and improve the body's acid-base status, which is compromised with aging.

Because muscle tissue activation is related to the resistance and the total amount of work performed, rest period lengths should be consistent with your goals for the program. Your medical or physical condition can also determine how much rest you should take. In some older adults (e.g., those with type 1 diabetes), gains in strength are the primary goal. Therefore, care must be taken to properly control the rest length between sets and exercises to prevent severe or intolerable metabolic stress. Tolerance of the workout in the context of progress toward specific goals is the key to optimizing workout quality. Rest period length plays a crucial role in this program design process.

Consistency Is the Key to Reaching Your Goals

Consistency is the foundation of success in reaching your fitness goals. With consistent effort, you will likely achieve your desired results. Here are just a few reasons why consistency is so crucial when it comes to fitness:

First, it allows you to make steady progress toward your goals. Your body gradually adapts and improves when you consistently exercise and eat healthily. You may not see dramatic results overnight, but over time, you will notice a significant difference in your strength, endurance, and overall health. This progress is much more sustainable than the yo-yo effect of starting and stopping an exercise routine.

Second, you develop healthy habits. Regular exercise becomes a part of your daily routine, making it easier to stick with over the long term. Additionally, when you eat healthily, you will be less likely to crave unhealthy foods and more likely to make good food choices. These healthy habits will make it easier to maintain your fitness level over time.

Third, you build confidence. When you see yourself progressing toward your fitness goals, you will feel more confident in your ability to achieve them. Additionally, you will feel better about yourself and your body when you are consistent with your exercise and healthy eating habits. This increased confidence can motivate you to continue working toward your goals.

Fourth, consistency helps you prevent injury. You are at a higher risk of injury when you jump into an intense workout or change your routine too quickly. By starting with a steady, moderate exercise routine and gradually increasing the intensity and duration, you will be less likely to get injured.

Fifth, it is crucial to staying motivated. When you have a regular workout routine, it becomes easier to track your progress and see the results of your efforts. This is a great motivator to keep going, especially when you don't feel like exercising. You will be less likely to feel guilty or discouraged when you indulge in an unhealthy treat.

But to be consistent, it is wise to set realistic goals. Setting unrealistic goals makes it easy to become discouraged and give up when you don't see immediate results. Additionally, being patient and persistent in working toward your goals is a significant accomplishment. It may take some time to see substantial results, but if you stick with it, you will get there.

It is also a good idea to track your progress. By keeping track of your exercise and eating habits, you can see where to adjust to stay on track. Additionally, as you progress, you can use this information to set new, more challenging goals.

In conclusion, consistency is the key to reaching your fitness goals. You can progress toward your desired results by consistently exercising and eating healthily. In short, consistency helps you develop healthy habits, build confidence, prevent injury, and stay motivated. So, remember to set realistic goals, be patient and persistent, and track your progress to stay consistent and achieve your fitness goals.

Key Takeaways

- When a senior's long-term strength training goal progresses toward higher levels of muscular strength, research supports the use of variation in the strength training program.

- Before starting any exercise, to determine training progress and personalize the program for yourself, you want to evaluate your strength, muscle endurance, functional ability, nutrition, and quality of life.

- Strength training programs must be designed and implemented to minimize the risk of injury and consider any limitations or restrictions a senior may have.

- Proper exercise technique is vital to safely implementing a strength training program.

- Vary the intensity and volume of your workout to ensure recovery, especially after workouts where significant muscle damage has occurred because of heavy resistances or high volumes.

- It is important to focus primarily on all major muscle groups over a week. You want to mix and match routines to build your plan.

CONCLUSION

"Strength does not come from winning. Your struggles develop your strengths. When you go through hardships and decide not to surrender, that is strength."

– Arnold Schwarzenegger

In choosing to read this book, you have taken the first step on a journey toward greater strength and vitality. As you can see, seniors can implement strength training safely and successfully. Even the frail and very sick elderly can gain benefits that will improve their quality of life. Muscle strength and power enhance everyday activities and quality of life, boosting many physiological characteristics, especially in the bones, muscles, and connective tissues.

Our discussion throughout this guide challenges common beliefs that traditional strength training is inappropriate for older people. Formal strength training for this population is effective if the program is properly designed and supervised and appropriately accounts for individual characteristics, such as clinical conditions and social, psychological, and economic considerations. Strength training is also important because it helps build and maintain muscle mass, improve balance and coordination, and increase energy levels. It can also reduce the risk of falls and fractures, improve physical and mental health, and help with activities of daily living. Another benefit has been shown to reduce symptoms of depression, improve sleep, and reduce the risk of developing chronic diseases such as heart disease and diabetes. Strength training for seniors is well on its way to being an accepted modality for fighting the aging processes and improving physiological function and performance among seniors.

The benefits for seniors are numerous and should not be overlooked. By following all the lessons and practicing all the simple but effective exercises we have covered in the *Strength Training for Seniors*, you can be on the path to rewriting your fitness journey as you age.

You will find the proper exercise in this guide if you want to improve your cardiovascular health, build muscle strength, or increase your flexibility and balance. Just make sure to start slowly and gradually increase your workouts' intensity. Also, always consult with your doctor before starting a new exercise program.

As the famous Chinese proverb says, "**The first thing to do is start. And the second is to continue**," so all you have to do now is to start. You already have the resources and information at your fingertips. Don't hesitate to go out there and use them.

Meanwhile, If you enjoyed the book, it would mean a lot to me if you could leave a review on Amazon with your kind feedback. As a new publisher, it requires many reviews for this book to be seen by others and I would love to reach as many as possible. Thank you so much for all your help.

I wish you the very best in your strength training journey!

To your success,

Linda Andrews

REFERENCES

Chiung-ju, L. (2009, July 8). *Progressive resistance strength training for improving physical function in older adults.*

Eldergym Fitness for Seniors. (2015). *Treatment for back pain for seniors - pelvic tilt.*

Eldergym Fitness for Seniors. (2016). *Overhead press.*

Elderly Gym Blog. (2023). *Knee strengthening exercises for seniors and the elderly.*

Fetters, K. A., & Esposito, L. (2020, September 30). *12 best equipment-free strength exercises for older adults.*

Freytag, C. (2021, October 07). *Basic strength training with good form.*

Kilroy, D. S. (2019, October 16). *Exercise plan for seniors.*

Koop, C. (2022, February 28). *Weight training for seniors: 3 basic exercises.*

Kutcher, M. (2020, October 1). *Stretching the quadriceps - made easy for seniors!*

Martin, M. (2021, November 7). *Chair squats.*

MasterClass. (2021, June 7). *Step-up exercise guide: how to do step-ups with perfect form.*

Melore, C. (2012, February 8). *Lifting weights for just 3 seconds a day can improve muscle strength.*

More Life Health Seniors. (2021). *15-minute strength workout for seniors.*

NCOA Blog. (2021, September 23). *10 reasons why hydration is important.*

NHS Inform Blog. (2022). *Warm-up and cool-down.*

Purdie, J. (2022, October 26). *What Is a Cool-down?*

Quinn, E. (2022, October 05). *19 bodyweight exercises to build strength.*

Ramsey, K. (2022, June 20). *8 knee strengthening exercises for seniors.*

SEO Blog. (2023). *Wall Push-ups.*

https://www.seniorexercisesonline.com/push.html.

Schoenfeld, B. J., Gorgic, J., Van Every, D. W., & Plotkin, D. L. (2021, February 22). *Loading recommendations for muscle strength, hypertrophy, and local endurance: a re-examination of the repetition continuum.*

Schrage, S. (2017, July 10). *Why strength depends on more than muscle.*
,

Seguin, R. A., Epping, J. N., Buchner, D. M., Bloch, R., & Nelson, M. E. (2002). *Growing stronger - strength training for older adults.*

Senior Lifestyle. (2023). *7 best exercises for seniors (and a few to avoid!).*

Steel Blog. (2021, December 11). *7 best back extension variations you can do at home.*

USC Verdugo Hills Hospital. (2022). *5 hand exercises to help you maintain your dexterity & flexibility.*

Velazquez, E. (2022). *The greatness of step-ups.*

Vokoun, R. (2021, July 13). *Why you should never skip your post-workout cool-down.*